When Infertility Books Are Not Enough:
Embracing Hope During Infertility

Betsy Herman

Printed in the United States of America

Cover Design: Rebekah Hauck

Cover and Author Photograph: Kim Baker / Chasing Sunsets

To every woman longing for a baby

CONTENTS

Prologue

Part 1: My Story

Part 2: My Spiritual Journey

Part 3: My Practical Suggestions

About the Author

Recommended Resources

Notes

Acknowledgements

Prologue

Tears well up in my eyes as I think of the correspondence that I've shared with women in the past few days as I complete this book.

Those words of encouragement from a mama who just gave birth to her first child: "One thing I have learned is that our baby is the baby God always intended us to have. It took ten years to meet her, and now that we are in this moment in time we know some of the reasons why it took so long…"

When I told an unmarried friend that this book is also for her: "I've waited so long for the blessing of a husband and children… it brought tears to my eyes to have a friend who stands with me."

No matter what the reason that you're not a mom yet, you are not alone. The reasons can be deeply personal: no husband, irregular menstrual cycles, or a failed adoption. Or the reasons can be completely unknown. Any of these can tempt us to shake our fist at God.

My own story consists of years filled with cycles of hope and disappointment. Right now my body reminds me that we didn't succeed at pregnancy this time and we won't be laying our eyes on our baby in nine months. I look toward Heaven with a mind filled with "WHY!?" questions for God.

Why, God? Why isn't this happening? Is it too much to ask You for a baby?

No, it's not too much for Him to handle, and it's not unreasonable for us to ask. However, in these years of waiting, I have learned so much more about the character of God – that He is in charge, and that He is for us and not against us. My faith is deeper. My capacity to hope has expanded, and God has given me grace for this season, a grace I never could have mustered up on my own.

I never expected to have trouble getting pregnant. Prior to getting married and trying to start a family, I would have said that infertility is one of the worst things I could imagine. Having experienced it firsthand, I can assure you that I wouldn't wish it on my worst enemy.

Let me take you through my journey, not so much focusing on the physical journey, but let me take you through the journey that happened within my soul throughout our years of being unable to conceive a baby. I want to describe the heart behind the matter – the emotional and spiritual side of this struggle. If you are having difficulty conceiving, or if you simply want to understand someone who is, or if you just want to read a story about a God who gives hope in discouraging circumstances, then keep reading.

Part 1 – My Story

Chapter 1 – I Just Want to Have a Baby

The LORD had closed her womb.
In her deep anguish
Hannah prayed to the LORD,
weeping bitterly.
1 Samuel 1:5 & 10

One afternoon not too long ago, I turned to my friend in the passenger seat of my car and asked, "What is your dream job?" She responded, "To be a wife and mom." This lovely woman is still asking God for a husband, and although she is a decade older than me, lives in another state, and has a different skin color than me, none of those differences matter. In fact, I hear that sentiment expressed often: recently from my single friend as she turned thirty, and from another young woman who has been married for several years and feels trapped in her career.

The more I talk to women, the more I realize how many of us share the same deeply rooted dream of primarily being wives and mothers. In a time and place where women can pursue nearly any career and go after any dream, I find that motherhood is one of the greatest desires of our hearts.

Yet some of us feel like this dream remains out of reach. Some wonder if marriage will ever happen, and some married women like myself wonder why starting a family seems to be so challenging.

Like so many others, one of my greatest dreams has always been to be a mother. My own mother was a stay-at-home mom and a wonderful role model – why would I want to pursue a career when

I could just take care of babies and hang out with kids all day? That desire never wavered through my teen years and into my college days.

I played with dolls until I was in my early teens. As a tot I had a life-sized doll named Rachel, who I loved, even though her fingers were chewed off by our dog. My favorite Cabbage Patch doll still lives in our guest room; his name is Damien. I enjoyed playing school with my siblings in our basement. Using our imagination, we transformed our backyard into the farm on which we worked. Often when we played house, I was the mother, and I had many, many children.

As a girl, I had a baby name book which I used to carefully name my dolls or fictional characters in stories I wrote. I made lists of names that I dreamed of naming my future children.

In my middle school years, I remember building houses with LEGOs and dreaming up the family that would live inside of them. Becoming an architect crossed my mind, because I loved drawing the floor plans for elaborate homes designed for a family with many children. When I was growing up, I dreamed of having fourteen children of my own one day. Eventually that number narrowed down to ten, then when I was in my twenties I would have said I'd like six children.

Now that I'm in my mid-thirties and have been married for a while, I would be happy to have any number of children! Although our plans could change, my husband Mike and I agree that one child would be a great start but two or three is our current goal. However, I regularly face the struggle of just wanting to be a mom, such a natural desire that seems so impossible since I have not been able to become pregnant yet.

As a teenager, I transitioned away from playing with dolls and started taking care of real babies and children, first in my own home and then babysitting for neighbors. As the oldest of four kids, I was given opportunities to babysit my siblings at a young age. At around nine or ten years old, I became a mother's helper for a family friend, and in the years following I began to babysit for our next-door-neighbors and other families that we knew. In my early teens, my mom and dad became foster parents, and I have happy memories of holding, feeding, and changing diapers of the little ones in our care. Some were certainly more challenging than others, but I loved the time with the babies.

In my high school English class, each student was required to create a resume. I suppose that our teacher hoped that those of us who didn't attend college would be prepared to start working. I had a handful of ambitions at that time – career aspirations that have never wavered. I wanted to be a wife and mother. I wanted to be a writer. I was open to being a missionary. And if those didn't work out, my dream career was to be a childcare provider. I found that high school resume several years ago, after finishing college and working in a variety of jobs. In my thirties, that old resume reminded me that my dream job was to care for children, so now I'm a full-time nanny. As I take care of other people's children I continue to dream of having my own little ones.

After graduating from high school, I spent a year doing missionary work in Panama. Living far from family, in another culture, and daily seeing people who lived in a simpler and more impoverished world was difficult. I grew up that year, however I also ended it feeling desperate for stability.

As my time in Panama reached an end, I struggled to know what to do with my life. At age nineteen I knew my long-term plan was to have a family of my own. I had no desire to pursue a serious career, so why would I need a college degree? Since I couldn't figure out what else to do in life, I headed off to a small Christian college in Tennessee.

Many clichés applied to college girls like me. "Are you going to college to get your M.R.S. degree?" Some young ladies made it their goal to get engaged before graduation with "a ring by spring!" I met lifelong friends during my college years, however I didn't meet my future husband. Even though I graduated a semester early and got a desk job right away, my passion was still family-oriented. I loved babysitting for little children and as I cared for and snuggled other people's babies, I dreamed of having my own.

3

I began working full-time immediately after graduating from college, and then finally got married. The time came when we were officially ready to start our family.

It would seem that motherhood should come easily for me: I loved children and wanted nothing else but to be a mom. However, that was not the case.

A year and a half into marriage, Mike and I began actively trying to conceive, and we found ourselves faced with month after month of disappointment. I would look down at my belly, plump with too many desserts, and empty of new life. Friends and acquaintances would greet me with "How are you?" but instead of making eye contact, I would watch their eyes steal a glance at my midsection to see if I looked pregnant.

Although I was not pregnant, women with the maternal glow and blooming bellies were everywhere. At the rare moment none of my close friends were pregnant, they had little ones in their arms. At church, at work, at the mall or Target, wherever I went, I was surrounded by new babies. Friends and relatives announced pregnancies one after the other. (One particular year, five of our cousins, my sister-in-law, and several close friends all had babies. Some then had another, all in the same amount of time we've been trying to have our first.)

Coworkers bragged about how quickly they conceived once stopping birth control, teenagers had babies that were not part of their plan, and it seemed that every woman in my church popped out their first kid within a year of the wedding. Looking around on a Sunday morning, it seemed that Mike and I were sitting in the center of an exceptionally fertile church in a very fertile world.

Mike and I had married on a beautiful November day, and eighteen months later we officially began trying to start our family. It was a significant moment. Not only were we both finally ready for a baby, but also the timing coincided with "our vacation of a lifetime." At the time we were stuck in jobs we didn't love, which only sweetened our time away. Having saved up our vacation time from work, we took off for three and a half weeks of traveling Europe.

Upon arrival in Germany, we rented a tiny Nissan and drove throughout the German countryside, then into Austria, Italy, Switzerland, and France before spending our final week with Mike's extended family in Lithuania. This was a glorious vacation! Sure, there were plenty of challenges such as navigating so many roads, cultures, and languages, but we planned for this to be our big getaway before having children. What can be more romantic than a glass of Italian wine, seeing historic cities and beautiful countrysides, and spending day and night with your love? Despite the fact that we had a fabulous trip, it was evident to me by the end of our travels that I had not become pregnant.

We'll give it another try, we told ourselves.

No success.

The months became years, filled with disappointment and tears. For me, the early months and years were the hardest. Maybe it's like other challenges in life: sometimes you get used to them. Sometimes the struggle simply makes you stronger. I recently trained for and ran my first half marathon. I haven't been much of a runner until this year, and the first time I ran more than three miles, it was a big deal. It was hard. Now, the challenge of running a long distance has gotten easier. Sure, it's still hard, but I'm used to it. I'm even getting good at it.

Although I don't want to get good at not being pregnant, I am grateful that through my circumstances I am becoming stronger. I have found myself filled with God's grace. I see His goodness even in this hardship. I realize that I am growing in faith, and I want to share this journey with you because I realize that I am not alone. God has infused my heart with hope and my desire is that by reading this, you will be encouraged, filled with hope, and able to face your circumstances with strength and grace.

Chapter 2 – First Comes Love

Love always hopes.
1 Corinthians 13:7

Even though my life-long dream has been to be a wife and mom, I wanted to do things in God's order, which meant getting married before pursuing motherhood. Well, I did strongly consider becoming a foster parent before I met my husband, but I was committed to saving sex for marriage (thankfully, so was Mike), and I wanted to follow God's leadership in dating.

For many years I dreamed of how my own story would play out. As I met various guys throughout my teenage and young adult years, I wondered, *Is he the one?* and *Is this the beginning of my love story?* Looking back, it's very clear that each of those guys were, in fact, not right for me.

It's hard to know the very beginning of a love story. Since my husband is a dozen years older than me, I like to say that the beginning of our love story was when God saw a basketball-loving, intelligent, introverted boy growing into a young man and God said, "Let Me make a helper suitable for him." Then He created me to one day be Mike's wife.

Although Mike had dated several women, he was steadfast in his desire to marry the woman God intended for him. I never dated anyone when I was a teenager. I wanted to, but the type of guy I was holding out for didn't cross my path often, and when he did, romance didn't happen. Like many other girls, I managed to have a whole lot of romance and wishful thinking in my head and heart, but not in my relationships. Although I wanted to find my special

7

someone when I was a teenager, I can now see the unfolding of God's plan in my life.

As a college student I was definitely on the lookout for Mr. Right. I didn't find him in college, and I didn't find him in my early twenties. It wasn't for lack of trying. It was difficult. I was lonely. I wanted to be married.

In college and into my twenties, I wallowed in self-pity and sadness that I was single. I wanted to be married and was very frustrated that life didn't seem to be going in that direction. I tried to hide my attitude of self-pity about singleness, but it was there. I cried easily and often. I am thankful that I have matured considerably. God has dealt with some major issues in my heart, so although I am still a passionate person, I am no longer as controlled by negative feelings.

Often I felt like God had forgotten about me. I would look around and see Him blessing others with fulfilled dreams, and I would wonder if He would ever answer my prayers. Even when I did not voice my struggle, several people in those years said to me that "God has not forgotten you."

In this season of desperately wanting to have children, I remember my wait for a husband. I remember the feelings of despair. The devil was whispering lies that I believed, such as thoughts of how God didn't care about me, or that He was leaving me to fend for myself. However, after seeing the faithfulness of God in providing such an amazing husband for me, now I can look forward with trust that God will also provide children.

Recently Jonah 2:8 (1984 NIV) caught my attention: "Those who cling to worthless idols forfeit the grace that could be theirs." Another translation (NKJV) says, "Those who regard worthless idols forsake their own mercy."

As I pondered this Scripture, I dug into a couple of commentaries on this verse in Jonah to understand this phrase better. The Matthew Henry commentary says that when they "forsake their own mercy" they turn their backs on their own happiness. The Chuck Smith commentary says that when we turn to anything other than embracing God we are essentially running from God.

He says it's as if we are fighting against a brick wall, therefore making it hard on ourselves instead of turning to God.

Marriage and children are valuable things, but when we turn them into idols, they're worthless idols. When I was desperately clinging to the idol of marriage, I wasn't walking through those years in my life with grace.

I did a lot of right things in the years when I was wanting to get married, but my heart was not at peace. Instead of embracing the God who loved me and wanted to bless me, I made the wait hard on myself.

My wait for children is similar to my wait for a husband. It's not in my control and I'm trying to trust God's ways and His timing. Since I waited while essentially beating a brick wall years ago, I don't really care to do that again. Having children is a good thing, but if it's my idol, it's a worthless idol, and if I cling onto that worthless idol, I'm giving up grace that could be mine. Now, instead of giving up that grace, I'm doing all I can to trust the God who is orchestrating my life.

So, while my wait for marriage wasn't always fun, it helped me to develop patience, trust, and faith. Through that process, I learned that God is looking out for me and that He will take care of me. There are many parallels between asking God for a husband and asking Him for a baby. Thankfully my previous experience of waiting for a husband built my faith and gave me the strength to look at my current circumstances and face my future and say, "God's timing is right."

Being single was hard. My friends were marrying one by one and I was a bridesmaid in three back-to-back weddings. I remember crying with sadness for myself when I could have been rejoicing for those getting engaged or married. Sure, I still had single friends, and we had fun. We were silly. We had serious moments where we dreamed of our futures and discussed what we were looking for in a spouse. Each of us was lonely and desiring marriage.

And I prayed. Family and friends were praying for me. I prayed some more. Then I got tired of praying.

"Did you just say that you got tired of praying?" Yes, I clearly remember one Sunday evening when I was about twenty-five. I went to a neighboring town to hear a visiting pastor who would be ministering at a church service. I was with my friend Sarah that night, and she turned to me at the end of the service and said, "I'm going to go ask him to pray for me to find a husband. Do you want to come and have him pray for you too?" I was quite fed up with my singleness at this point, so my cynical response as I stayed in my chair was, "No thanks. If God hasn't heard me by now, what's another prayer going to matter?"

I didn't ask for prayer that night.

Not too long after that church service, I began to feel even more desperation for marriage and openness toward dating someone I didn't know well. The turning point where I started getting serious about getting married was around the time I turned twenty-six. Although it might sound young, many of my peers were already married and starting families, and I knew that I just wanted to be a wife and mom. I was tired of sitting around waiting for something to happen, and I realized that where I was and what I was doing was not getting me any closer to marriage.

One unusual week that winter, I opened my email to discover messages from two women I knew from church who were inquiring if I would be interested in meeting men they knew. Completely independently of each other they were trying to set me up with someone. In my younger years, I would have freaked out and been too nervous about meeting a strange guy and might have thought, *How could this possibly be from God if this is a person trying to set me up! Isn't God supposed to be my matchmaker?*

I gave both women permission to give my information to the guys. The local guy was apparently too shy to ever call me. When I heard the news that he had died in a tragic car accident a year later, I was grateful that we had not dated.

The other guy ended up being my first boyfriend. Jason and I emailed, then called, then met in person a few times. He lived in another state so seeing each other required travel. Although we called it "dating" there wasn't much to our relationship. After holding on desperately to the idea that he was "the one," I finally determined that he really wasn't all that interested in me or committed to me, so I ended the relationship. Although I often view that relationship as a waste of my time, I also see it as one of the things that motivated me to move to a new state, where I would meet the love of my life.

After the breakup, feeling ready for a fresh start and a new environment, and with much prayer, I decided it was time to move, and it's a move I do not regret.

So one April day in 2007, with the help of friends, I packed my life into a U-Haul and drove over the mountains to a new state. I quickly settled into my job and the townhouse that I shared with my sister, and I soon found a church... one that had a large and active singles group, of course. There I met new faces and, I will confess, I was definitely on the lookout for My Future Husband. I enjoyed getting to know new people and I made some lasting friendships in that group. However, while I was busy looking for My Future Husband within my social group, I almost missed him!

That summer, as I was enjoying being the new girl in town, I had a significant moment in prayer. One night at the church prayer meeting we paired up with someone nearby to pray for each other. In one of these moments, I thought to myself, *I wish I could just ask this woman to pray for me to find a husband!* I didn't feel comfortable presenting such a request to a random woman at church, but the thought lingered with me for a few days. That week I thought about my self-consciousness in sharing that request, and I remembered Sarah who went forward at an altar call with that very same prayer request. *Hmm*, I thought to myself, *she confidently asked God for a husband, and I refused because I was tired of praying about it. Now she's married... and I'm not.*

I wonder if my life would have turned out differently if I had overcome my fear of what people thought and humbly asked people to pray that I would get married. I'm not sure I would have gotten married any sooner, but I imagine that by sharing my struggle I would have walked through my wait with more grace and peace.

In the middle of that summer, I had been living in my new state for several months, and I was sitting in my old blue station wagon in a grocery store parking lot. I remember that I sensed God giving me the words to pray. I scribbled this prayer onto a piece of paper: "God I ask that in this hour, in this city, in this church, in this season I would find my husband, that I wouldn't be ashamed to ask or receive, that You, Lord, would hear and answer the cries of my heart."

My faith surged and I knew deep in my heart that things were about to change. Not long after that, a gentleman expressed interest in me, but his interest fizzled quickly. I felt confused, but I believed that prayer I had prayed. Deep inside, I sensed that breakthrough was coming.

Chapter 3 – Then Comes Marriage

The Lord God said,
"It is not good for the man to be alone.
I will make a helper suitable for him."
Genesis 2:18

One evening in late August 2007, I joined the single's group at my church to watch a minor league baseball game. It turned out that we couldn't get tickets to the sold-out game, so we ended up eating dinner at a nearby restaurant. Toward the end of the meal I found myself chatting with a guy from the group whom I had never met or even noticed before. When the conversation ended, I went on about my business... and little did I know that for the next four months, while I wondered where My Future Husband was, that very guy was trying to have a follow-up conversation with me!

Mike and I would mostly see each other across the enormous sanctuary during the Wednesday night prayer service at our church. We attended a large church so we rarely crossed paths on Sundays, although I could see him from where I normally sat. The Wednesday evening gatherings had fewer people and, to his dismay, I would often tiptoe in late and slip out early as I was exhausted from my busy life and stressful job. On the rare days that I stayed until the end of the service, Mike would find me huddled together with girlfriends (complaining about the lack of available men, I'm sure), which made me hard to approach.

Although I didn't realize that he wanted to talk to me, I did know that his name was Mike, and as time went on that fall I often found myself watching him during church. Even when he wasn't looking in my direction, I would notice him. I could tell he was at least several years older than me, and I would ask myself, *Betsy! Why are you noticing this guy with gray hair?* All I knew about him was that he was a faithful member at our church and I liked watching him pray and worship the Lord. That was enough for my interest in him to grow.

Throughout this time I was doing a lot of praying. God was showing me that new beginnings were just around the corner. I was working through feelings of rejection from the past. I remember crying on Christmas Day as I drove by myself back to my townhouse. I felt so alone after the festivities. I was tired of the loneliness of not having a husband, and again I asked the Lord to bring my future spouse into my life. That same week I found myself thinking about Mike. I didn't know him, but I did ask God for an opportunity to get to know him. That opportunity was about to come faster than I expected.

Less than a week after asking God for a chance to get to know Mike, it was time for Wednesday night prayer. We had a rather small group at church, and we met in a smaller room than usual. I arrived late and as I approached the locked door, Mike opened it for me and greeted me with, "Hello, Betsy."

He knows my name! He said hello! I'm sure those thoughts distracted me for the rest of the prayer time. None of my girlfriends were there that night, I was on the far side of the room from the door, and Mike walked over to talk to me afterward. Basically he cornered me. After all, he had been trying since late summer to talk to me, and it was January at this point.

Mike struck up a conversation that led to, "So, would you like to go for coffee sometime?" Poor guy, he didn't know how much I like coffee and that he'd be buying me coffee for the rest of our lives! The suggestion to go out for coffee evolved into lunch plans the following Sunday.

That Saturday night was the eve of my fourth first date. (Obviously, I didn't go on many dates.) Like all the other nights before a date, it was a sleepless night. Even though I was tired, we met at the café near my townhouse after church, where we talked… and talked… and talked, to the point where Mike lost his voice. We found common ground in our families and similar hopes for the future. When we left the café, he gave me a gift he had bought for me on a business trip to Africa the month before. It was a little blue beaded basket – and I loved it! It was a good feeling to know that he had been thinking of me before we really even knew each other!

I went home that day and put my Internet stalking skills to use. I discovered that Mike had just turned 40 a month before. My thoughts for the next day went something like this: *40! Why not 39, God? 40 sounds so old, I'm only 28!* Well, as Mike and I continued to communicate and see each other that week, I got over the age difference pretty quickly. This was a man I wanted to get to know. My advice for people who meet someone who is different from what they always dreamed of is this: sometimes giving up preconceived notions can be a very good move! This principle also applies to starting a family – giving up my own ideas of when and how will release me to be open to God's timing and His ways.

Although I was young when we began dating, I had been comparing myself to my closest friends who were already married with children, so I felt like a leftover. Several weeks into our relationship, Mike said something that brought healing to my heart. He said he went home from our first date with a sense that he had found a hidden treasure.

One of the most important things that I have come to realize in recent years is that many of the thoughts I embrace are not truth, and they are not from God. These harmful thoughts could come from my own mind, emotions, and soul, or they could be spoken to me by the devil. Beginning to see circumstances through the perspective of God's heart toward me, and not simply seeing things based on my feelings or the lies from the enemy of my soul has changed my life.

Four weeks into our dating relationship, Mike and I took a hike together. It was a warm winter day and we hopped along some rocks in a quiet river. Mike's rock-hopping skills confirmed that he was strong, athletic, confident, and all around the kind of guy that I wanted in my life. Compared to other guys I had hiked with who were too cocky or too clumsy, Mike seemed just right. I remember thinking, *If he asked me to marry him right now, I'd say yes.* At that moment I slipped and fell into the water... and he didn't propose for another five months.

During our dating days, from January through June, we met each other's families, enjoyed some fun dates like going to the theater and out to eat, took a few trips to visit family and friends, and had lots of serious conversations. While we were dating we talked through a lot of serious issues so that if we decided to get married we could move forward. Our months of dating certainly had some stressful times, and I admit that I shed many tears as I tried to figure out how to relate to this new person.

In late June 2008, Mike felt that he had heard from the Lord clearly enough that it was right for us to be married. (I had decided back in January.) We realized that my dad was getting ready to leave the country for a couple of weeks, so Mike talked with my dad on a Friday evening. Saturday was the first time Mike mentioned engagement rings to me. (I had been trying to not get my hopes up prematurely, and it was difficult!) Then on Sunday he suggested we look at rings together. We visited several jewelers so I could figure out the style I loved, and when I went home that night, I suspected that he would propose soon, perhaps as soon as the following weekend. I didn't know that he had returned to the store and bought my ring that very same day!

The following evening, I headed off with some girls to a going-away party for a friend. I told Mike that I thought I might be back at my apartment around nine p.m. My friends and I took our time at that good-bye party, although had I been aware of Mike's plan, I would have hurried back!

Without my knowing, he had made a reservation at our favorite restaurant and bought me the most beautiful roses he could find – this was my first bouquet of roses. I returned from the party closer to 10, and although Mike had to cancel the dinner reservation, as we sat in my living room talking that night, he asked me to marry him. Although I don't remember his exact words, I do remember saying "Yes!" I know without a doubt we made the right decision and that I married the very best one for me! Over and over again since that night I have thought about how there is no one I'd rather be taking this journey with than Mike. He continually encourages me and helps me to grow as a person and as a Christian.

Four months after our engagement we were married. After our rehearsal dinner we had a "toasting party" where we invited family and close friends to make a toast and share a word of encouragement with us. At the end of that sweet evening I told our guests that we were glad the wedding day had finally arrived. "Mike might have waited longer, but I waited harder," I said. Those who walked with me through that wait knowingly agreed. I believe this is true: the best and most treasured things in life are worth waiting for.

Just as it was hard for me to wait for my husband, it has been hard to wait for babies to come. I do not wait well by nature. I'm type-A and I like to have a plan then make it happen. I feel anxious, I think about the future, I make plans and wonder why they aren't working out. Yet while I was waiting for a husband I learned so much about waiting, trusting God, and releasing my grip on how I thought things would happen. I feel like this battle for fertility is round two of that same test: can I wait? Can I walk through life with grace while I wait? Will I trust the God to whom I have dedicated my life?

As I wrote my love story of how I came to be Mrs. Herman, I remember many tears and prayers during my wait. I felt sad and lonely. I didn't like the wait: it seemed long and it was surely hard.

Then I remember the specific prayer in July 2007 that God "would hear and answer the cries of my heart." For reasons that are God's alone, that hot Sunday afternoon was the moment God broke through, essentially saying to me: "It's time." As I await my babies, I am writing this, believing I will one day have a breakthrough and a hope fulfilled. It is so important to look back and see that God was faithful to answer my prayer request about getting married. Even though it wasn't exactly when or how I expected, God's answer has been so very right. Knowing that He was faithful in the past strengthens my belief that He is able to answer my prayers in the future according to His plans.

Inscribed in our wedding program from November 2008 is this Scripture: *"You have granted him his heart's desire and have not withheld the request of his lips." Psalm 21:2*

That's God. He might not do things in our timing or exactly how we would have scripted them, but He is the one who fulfills those deep longings within us.

Chapter 4 – Then Comes the Baby… or Not?

For You created my inmost being;
You knit me together in my mother's womb.
I praise You because I am fearfully and wonderfully made;
Your works are wonderful,
I know that full well.
Psalm 139:13–14

Although my primary focus is on the emotional and spiritual journey in the fertility struggle, I also want to share briefly about the physical and medical side of this experience. Everyone is different, and our personal lives and health are varied. Please keep in mind that this book is not intended to provide any medical advice; I am simply sharing how the process of seeking medical help has gone for us.

I've always considered myself to be relatively healthy and in a reasonable weight range. I presumed that because I was healthy and my family members had no known problems conceiving, then I would be fine. I also assumed this about Mike, so why would we have any issues?

I was 28 and Mike was 40 when we married, then a year and a half into our marriage, we began trying for a baby. Both of us were virgins when we married, so we didn't have to worry about past history in that area of our lives.

My menstrual cycles have always been very predictable and right on time, if not early. They were usually accompanied by severe cramps, but I assumed that regular cycles would mean normal fertility. In our first year and a half of marriage we used hormonal birth control for a period of time, and then we used natural family planning for some of the time, which is my preferred option.

After six months of trying to get pregnant without success, I scheduled a doctor's appointment with an OB/GYN. She ordered some bloodwork which came back "just fine!" and the doctor recommended that I drink an occasional glass of red wine and try to relax. If only it were that easy.

I felt very conflicted during the first couple of years of trying to conceive – I believed that God could and would bring us a baby – and felt like taking fertility medications would be attempting to force God's hand and manipulate His timing. As we have thought, prayed and researched in these past few years, I have reached a few conclusions as to my own personal stance on fertility treatments. I realize that many people have different perspectives on what sort of (if any) fertility treatments to pursue, so this is strictly my opinion.

I want to live my life in a posture of surrender to God, believing that He creates new life in His timing. Therefore, Mike and I prayerfully pause to consider any new options in fertility treatment before taking a step. If there is an underlying physical issue that hinders a couple from conceiving, then I think that it is wise to treat that medical condition. This is best done with an attitude of surrender to God's will.

However, I personally am not very attracted to in-vitro fertilization (IVF). This fertility treatment involves stimulating the woman's ovaries with hormones then retrieving multiple eggs at once. In a lab, those eggs are fertilized with her husband's sperm unless there is a need for donor eggs or sperm. These embryos grow for several days in a lab, then are transferred back to the mother's womb, hopefully resulting in pregnancy. This method is costly and controversial. However, while writing this book, I have encountered many people who have pursued IVF as the means by which to have babies.

I believe that life begins the moment that an egg and sperm meet. IVF may involve tiny lives (fertilized eggs) being lost during the process. Some people prefer that their child be formed in the womb instead of a lab, but ultimately God is the one who creates new life, whether it is in a womb or in a lab. This is a highly debatable topic, and not desiring to stir up controversy, I simply want to say that IVF does not really appeal to me personally. My reasons include the ethical dilemma, the high cost, and the physical toll it takes on a woman's body as she must be injected with many hormones throughout the process.

Throughout our first couple of years we tried over-the-counter ideas such as supplements. I read books about fertility and researched the most optimal ways to get pregnant. I faithfully charted my cycle by taking my morning temperature, monitoring my cervical fluid, and being aware of other signs throughout each month. An excellent resource to learn about monitoring the fertility cycle is the book *Taking Charge of Your Fertility* by Toni Weschler[1].

When more than a year of trying without conception had passed by, my doctor at the time gave me a prescription for Clomid, a common fertility medicine that stimulates ovulation. I had been using ovulation tests for many months, and based on the tests and my fertility charts, I knew that I was ovulating. Realizing that Clomid increases the likelihood of multiple births (especially since this was around the time when Mike was beginning graduate school), we didn't feel like Clomid was the right approach for us, so I never filled the prescription.

We moved to Virginia where, by the Hand of Providence, we stumbled upon an OB/GYN practice that happened to be Catholic and therefore shared our conservative perspective. I called to make an appointment and mentioned our struggle to conceive, so the receptionist scheduled me to see the fertility specialist.

Dr. Lorna Cvetkovich, whom we call Dr. C, has been incredibly supportive. She is an expert in Natural Family Planning and overcoming infertility. She sees fertility from a faith-based perspective, which we appreciate. Upon our first visit, Mike and I told her about our medical history and discussed our years of trying to conceive. She suggested several tests, including a semen analysis for Mike and a test for me to see if my fallopian tubes were blocked.

This test is called a hysterosalpingogram (HSG). In this test, the specialist inserts dye into the uterus and simultaneously takes x-rays of the uterus and fallopian tubes to show whether or not the fallopian tubes are open. For many women this is a very painful procedure. I remember it hurting, but not being any worse than my usual menstrual cramps. It was an uncomfortable and invasive procedure to say the least. However, I was relieved at the end of it when the technician turned the screen around and showed me an image of my uterus and healthy-looking fallopian tubes.

When Mike's tests came back normal and my HSG was clear, Dr. C commented that I might have endometriosis. She suggested that I have a laparoscopic surgery to determine if I have it and, if necessary, to clean it out. Although this disease is hard to detect without surgery, my family history and painful menstrual cramps indicated that this might be an issue for me, so we were willing to proceed.

Endometriosis is when the lining of the uterus (the endometrium) grows outside of the uterus. This is a non-cancerous growth, but it can negatively affect the reproductive system and cause pain. During menstruation, the endometrium outside the uterus also bleeds, causing scar tissue and very painful cramping. According to the Mayo Clinic website, one-third to one-half of women with endometriosis have difficulty getting pregnant.

So, in April 2013, I had a quick outpatient laparoscopic surgery in which the doctor found and removed some endometriosis. Unfortunately she discovered the largest quantity clustered around one ovary and my ureter (the tube that carries urine from the kidney to the bladder). She didn't want to proceed in operating so close to the ureter without the assistance of the urologist, so a second surgery was scheduled.

Two months later I had a major conventional surgery involving a five inch incision and two nights in the hospital. The first week of recovery was tough, but within a couple of months I had bounced back to normal. When pregnancy didn't happen soon after the surgery, Mike and I agreed to try medication to assist my fertility.

Under the care of Dr. C, I began taking Tamoxifen, which is technically a breast cancer drug, although it works in a similar way to Clomid. It is friendlier to the cervical fluids and has a lower chance of multiple eggs being released, so we felt comfortable with this decision.

Also, while charting my fertility cycles, I discovered that my luteal phase, which is the time between ovulation and menstruation, was rather short. A normal luteal phase is around twelve to fourteen days long; mine are often closer to ten days. My periods typically come twenty-six days apart, meaning that if a sperm and egg are forming an embryo, it might not have enough time to successfully implant in the uterus before the uterus begins to shed the lining (menstruation).

Believing that life begins the moment that the egg is fertilized, and recognizing that my body was very likely losing fertilized eggs due to menstruation, Mike and I realized that tiny embryos – our much-wanted babies – are possibly being formed and lost. If that is happening, we might have many tiny children in Heaven.

After about six months of taking Tamoxifen monthly and being monitored by Dr. C, we agreed to switch to another similar medication called Femara. She also prescribed Prometrium, which is a synthetic form of progesterone, as a supplement after ovulation. This treats Luteal Phase Defect (a short luteal phase) and it has helped to lengthen my luteal phase, allowing more time for an embryo to implant. Women who take Prometrium during their luteal phase often take it throughout the first trimester to support the pregnancy and to help prevent miscarriage.

Most months, despite medications, my cycles are short. On those rare occasions when it's longer than 27 days, I face a daily battle of emotion as I speculate whether or not I could be pregnant. At the time of writing, I have never had a positive pregnancy test. I buy ovulation test strips and pregnancy test strips in bulk. I'm well acquainted with peeing into little plastic cups and having a needle stuck into my arm. Throughout these years I have had a lot of bloodwork to test one hormone level or another. I can usually predict what the nurse will say when I receive a phone call with my test results: "Your hormones look great!" I usually want to respond by pointing out that, "Well, obviously something is not great!"

My specialist, Dr. C, has been one of our biggest cheerleaders. Never has she said that it looks like we won't get pregnant. She has suggested new ideas or prescribed new medications, and every time I walk out of her office, I leave with a sense of hope that maybe one day soon I will become pregnant. We appreciate her perspective and her optimism!

I share all of this to say that medical intervention can be helpful, but medicine, surgery, and spending thousands of dollars does not guarantee a baby. The Creator of life is the answer – He is the only one who can bring about a new life inside a womb. Some pregnancies seem more miraculous than others – some are against all hope and against all odds – but every one of us was formed by God Himself. He is the One we should look to when we want offspring.

Psalm 139:13–16 reminds us that God creates new life within a mother's womb and verse 16 states, "All the days ordained for me were written in Your book before one of them came to be." He knows the specific day that new life will begin, and even though we have chosen to use medical assistance, we trust and believe that God is the One who will create new life within my womb.

Chapter 5 – Miracle Babies

She who was said to be barren is in her sixth month.
For nothing is impossible with God.
Luke 1:36–37

In these years that Mike and I have been trying to start a family, several women I know have given birth after it seemed impossible. Nothing compares to the joy of a long-awaited baby being born! As I have observed these friends in their years of trying to conceive and throughout their pregnancies and into life with their new babies, my faith has been strengthened. If God can do it for them, He can do it for us!

Debra

The first woman I'll call "Debra" to protect her privacy. We attended the same church, where we both met our husbands. We were married the same year, and I remember the day that a mutual friend told me that Debra was pregnant. I knew immediately that this was a long-awaited baby and couldn't wait to hear the full story.

Several months later I attended her baby shower. Like most mothers-to-be, Debra glowed with happiness at her shower. As the guests gathered for the opening of the gifts, Debra took a moment to share her story.

She had married at age forty to a widower who already had grown children as well as young grandchildren. As a career-oriented woman, she was not certain that she would adjust to the demands that children would require. However, once she was married and spent time with her stepchildren and grandbabies, she felt reminded that she would never experience a child calling her "mommy," that she didn't fall into the "mommy club," and would never be a mother of a bride. She realized that she would miss out on aspects of womanhood that we are specifically designed for. She began to feel a stronger desire to become a mother.

She described that for about eighteen months they tried to conceive. It was a challenging journey of hope and disappointment, carrying on with life, and celebrating with friends' babies while longing for her own. Only a few people knew that they were hoping for a child, and Debra describes that experience as very private and painful.

After a year of trying passed by, they saw a fertility specialist, who initially was optimistic until Debra's test results came back with bad news. According to the doctor, the only thing that could be done was in-vitro fertilization, and because Debra was 43 at the time, pregnancy would require donor eggs. The doctor also felt that the likelihood of her actually getting pregnant was slim, as he diagnosed her with age-related infertility.

This news devastated Debra. She describes how she felt that the term "infertility" became a loaded word, filled with pain, longing, and shame. She clearly recognized that becoming a mother in any form was a privilege and not a right. Motherhood is a special gift from God.

At her baby shower, and in the detailed story which she shared with me recently, Debra describes that after this doctor's appointment she had to make some decisions. First, she consciously chose to put her trust in God and leave it up to Him. Secondly, she chose to believe that God gave her the desire to be a mommy, and that He will fulfill it according to His will and purpose. Thirdly, she chose to cling to the prophetic words and visions of pregnancy and motherhood that had been shared with her, including a specific word having to do with the month of June (but did not say June of which year).

When June 2010 came and went and she was not yet pregnant, she felt extremely disappointed, however she says that she acknowledged that God's timing is perfect and that His plan would triumph.

Together with her husband, a decision was made to not give up on having a baby, yet to wait until the end of June 2011 before pursuing in-vitro fertilization. She chose to apply her faith and to put her hope in God. In May of that year, she was facing work-related problems and feelings of disappointment over not being pregnant. She shared that one morning she awakened at five o'clock, and when she couldn't fall back asleep she made some tea and poured her heart out to the Lord. She told Him that she couldn't go on, that she was out of energy, hope, and emotional strength.

The Holy Spirit spoke clearly to her, saying, "Don't give up now, you can see the end of the line, the winning line is in front of you, just keep going and keep moving forward." She replied, "Okay, Lord, I'll hold on, but after June, I give up, I'm done".

As she stood before friends and family at her baby shower the following year, she described that her faith had been renewed in that moment as she knew that the Lord had heard her cries! That June, she and her husband conceived a baby with no medical intervention. This was the month before they intended to pursue fertility treatments. After the doctors said it was highly unlikely that she would become pregnant due to her age, God did it!

In the last days of June she felt like she might be pregnant, and on the Fourth of July she took a home pregnancy test which was positive! Doctors confirmed it two weeks later and Debra's heart was filled with joy that she was going to be a Mommy, not only a stepmom and a grandmommy, but a Mommy!

At her baby shower she shared with us: "My God heard my prayer, He fulfilled the prophetic words and visions seen, and He is giving me beauty for ashes. I am so thankful! I pray that, as you face your own challenges and uncertainties, that you will take hope in mine... God did a miracle for me. He made a way in the desert, and He gave me the desire of my heart! May He also do it for you!"

Her pregnancy was easy, and her baby boy wasn't eager to leave the cozy womb, so she ended up having a Cesarean-section. However, all went well, and today as I write, Debra's son is an active, happy, and tall almost three-year-old. She wrote to me that, "God has truly given us beauty for ashes. He has made my hope complete. Whenever I am faced with difficulty and hoping for something good to come, I look at my son and recognize the sovereignty and goodness of God."

Many, many, miracle babies have been born in recent years, and I'm convinced that more are yet to come. When I think about her story, as I often do, I see that God can enable a woman to have a healthy pregnancy after doctors have said it's impossible. He is not held back by age, diagnosis, or any other circumstances. Debra's story continually reminds me that "nothing is impossible with God!"

Mandy

When Mandy announced her pregnancy last year, I was thrilled. These days, nothing compares to the joy I feel when someone has a baby after years of waiting and trying!

Mandy and I had attended the same church in Tennessee briefly before I moved away, but we didn't know each other personally. Since we had many mutual friends, we ended up becoming Facebook friends, and it was through social media that I learned that she was contending for a baby. She boldly proclaimed that God would make it happen! (And He did!)

When I was in her town, I finally met Mandy in person at a wedding just a few months ago, and since then we have talked so that I could hear her entire story.

When Mandy was only twelve years old, she was told that she wouldn't be able to have children due to severe endometriosis and ovarian cysts. She had surgery for these conditions as a sixth-grader, and doctors confirmed a few years later after her second surgery that they were pretty sure that she wouldn't be able to have babies.

Mandy still dreamed of becoming a mommy. Despite the doctors' predictions, Mandy became pregnant with her first child at age nineteen. Although she faced many challenges at the time, she carried that pregnancy and now has a teenage daughter. A few years later she met and married her husband Jason, who was the children's pastor at their church at that time. He has since adopted her firstborn.

Since she had a young child already, Mandy and Jason wanted to have babies right away. However, before their wedding day, Mandy heard the Lord speak to her as He has done many times. He said that she would have to contend for the seed of her husband. The Lord also promised Mandy that she would have a little girl and then a little boy.

Within their first year of marriage, she miscarried twice, and during their first seven years of marriage, they had a total of nine miscarriages. This devastated their family of three.

In the summer of 2010 after the final miscarriage, Mandy prayed that the Lord would close her womb until His perfect timing for her baby. He did, and she didn't become pregnant until more than two years later.

Between the eighth and ninth miscarriages, Mandy began seeing a new doctor. She was diagnosed with Protein C disorder, which is being treated with baby aspirin. She was prescribed Metformin to treat Polycystic Ovary Syndrome (PCOS). She then had surgery to clean up the lining of her uterus which had been damaged from many miscarriages.

After Mandy's ninth miscarriage, the doctor really wanted to help Mandy find a way to have a healthy pregnancy. She discovered that Mandy had a fibroid in the back of her uterus, where it would be difficult to operate. This doctor listened as Mandy described what was happening with her body. One day, about a year after the ninth and final miscarriage, Mandy was at her doctor's office and the physician stepped out of the room for a moment to research a potential treatment for her. She then prescribed Mandy with Prometrium. Mandy felt certain that she had a Luteal Phase Defect, and Prometrium is a synthetic form of progesterone, used to lengthen the luteal phase and support the developing baby during the first trimester. After taking this for nine months, her cycles were healthier and the doctor encouraged her that in a few more months it would be time to try for a miracle baby.

Not long after that, when her period didn't come on time, Mandy took a pregnancy test and was disappointed to see the single line. Her daughter, 14 at the time, said "I know you're pregnant, Mom!" She pulled the test out of the trash, moved toward a brighter light, and there WAS a second line!

Despite a lot of sickness throughout her pregnancy, Mandy carried that baby to full-term, and her baby girl just celebrated her first birthday this fall. Like many others, Mandy has reminded me that God's timing is perfect. She says that "it's not about us, because God is looking at the bigger picture."

When Mandy's youngest miracle baby was nine months old, we met face-to-face at a wedding. That weekend I spent some time hearing Mandy's story and holding that precious child. I walked away from our conversation encouraged spiritually: Mike and I had already determined that having a baby from my womb was the direction in which God was guiding us. Having a similar medical condition of a short luteal phase, I felt encouraged that Mandy felt that taking the progesterone supplements helped her become pregnant.

What impresses me the most about Mandy is her bold faith. In the season when she was hoping and trying to conceive, she was confident enough to post her prayers on Facebook. Now, using an app called TimeHop, she receives updates of what she wrote on that particular day years ago. In October 2014 Mandy wrote on Facebook, "I love being reminded of my faith walk in regards to seeing our miracles come forth. I don't remember posting about it so many times, but my faith gets a little jolt every time I see one of these pop up!" With this statement she referenced her post exactly four years earlier: "I speak life to my womb in Jesus name, and I thank and praise You Father, in faith, that our miracle babies are on their way!"

Mandy spoke life to her womb and after years of believing that God could do it, He did it. Understanding the power of the tongue and the authority given by Jesus, Mandy spoke forth what was to come. Then eventually, new life was formed inside of her, a pregnancy was carried to completion, and a miracle baby was born. After seeing what God has done for her thus far, I will not be surprised to hear that she is pregnant again, and this time with a boy.

Michelle

I met "Michelle" (whose name I'm changing for privacy) a few years ago when we attended a ministry training event. We were riding in the backseat of a friend's car, and before the trip ended, we discovered that we both wanted to have a baby but were not having success. Like me, she was comfortable telling people of her desire to have more children. At the time, she had two little boys entering into kindergarten and first grade.

When I met Michelle, she had been trying to have a baby for about four years. She says that her journey of trying to conceive was the greatest test of faith she has ever experienced. As newlyweds, she and her husband were given a prophetic word by a pastor that they would be very fertile. Despite that being the word of the Lord for this couple, they learned that they had to fight for their fertility.

In her years of trying to conceive, Michelle had several close friends in a similar fight for babies. Yet she remembers the emotions and the frustration of watching some couples have babies one after another, while she and her best friend were desperately asking God for more children, and finding themselves waiting.

One Sunday morning, a pastor at her church preached about the passage in Esther 4:14 where Esther's uncle says to her, "You were born for such a time as this." This pastor explained that God had specific purposes for the times his own children were born – that the Lord had already prepared in advance the people they would meet, the world events they would be part of, and the specific moments in which God intended to use them. Michelle left the service that day realizing that it wasn't just about her getting pregnant, it was about what God had planned for her child.

Michelle believed that she and her husband would have a daughter. People had dreams about her holding her newborn girl. Although there were days when she cried and cried because of her desire for a baby, she felt like it would eventually happen.

During her difficult wait for a baby, she began to see the toll that it was taking on her marriage. She realized that trying to conceive was very hard on their relationship because of the emotional pull on her. As women who want a baby, it's on our minds all the time. Hormones and periods, and the desire to mother and nurture are difficult to escape. Most husbands would agree that it's not on their minds all the time; it's not a burning desire. Her husband had a lot of job-related stress, which was hard on their marriage. At times she found herself reluctant to be intimate because intimacy was so closely associated with the disappointment of not being pregnant.

She came across a book called *The Respect Dare: 40 Days to a Deeper Connection with God and Your Husband* by Nina Roesner[1]. This is a resource written by a woman who was having a tough time with the biblical concept of submission. As Michelle and a small group of women worked through this book, taking steps to grow in respect to both God and their husbands, her marriage improved. Communication got better, and she discovered that doing something worthwhile during the wait made the time go by more enjoyably.

Although she was regularly seen by her OB/GYN, Michelle and her husband never visited a fertility specialist. They felt that in their early years of marriage they had tried to be in charge of the timing of their children too much, so they didn't want to interfere with God's timing.

Then, in 2012, after five years of trying to have a baby, her period was late and she took a pregnancy test one Sunday night. It was positive. She and her husband were delighted, and told their young sons about it since those boys had also been in prayer for a baby to come.

She called her doctor first thing in the morning, and went in for a confirmation of pregnancy. She found out that she was due on December 26 and felt excitement that God would give them such a gift. However, by Wednesday she began bleeding, and it was confirmed by the doctor to be a miscarriage.

Her little boys had questions: "Why would God take the baby on to Heaven?" Those were the same questions that Michelle and her husband were asking; some of the same questions that they'll ask God when they get to Heaven one day.

Michelle went home from the doctor and laid on her bed where she let the tears flow. Eventually that afternoon she knew she would need to get up and continue with life. Part of her wanted to keep going so that she could try again, as she still had hope that a baby would come.

Months went by, and no pregnancy came. That Christmas was especially difficult as Michelle was remembering the baby that had been due the next day.

The day after Christmas, returning home from a family gathering, Michelle cried as her husband drove down the interstate. During the festivities, family members had forgotten about the significance of that day for Michelle. As they drove, billboards with giant faces of babies advertising the labor and delivery department at the local hospital only intensified the reminder of the baby she had lost. She felt hurt and frustrated that her best friend was the only one to remember that date. She wondered, "Will Christmas always feel like this?"

But her friend was not the only one to remember.

Several months later, in timing that can only be orchestrated by a redemptive and loving Creator, Michelle discovered that she was again pregnant. She typed some dates into an online due date calculator and discovered that once again, exactly a year after her miscarriage, she was expecting a baby on December 26. Her sweet baby girl was born two days after Christmas that year!

Upon hearing these stories and writing this chapter, I climbed into my bed and said to my husband that now I feel even more of a sense that God will also give us a miracle baby. He has proven that He can do anything, with or without medical help, whether it seems possible or not.

Part 2 – My Spiritual Journey

Chapter 6 – It's Not Easy, Yet God is Good

How long must I wrestle with my thoughts
and day after day have sorrow in my heart?
Psalm 13:2

I didn't call my mom this past Mother's Day. I love my mom and I'm thankful for her, but I'm also grateful that she doesn't have major expectations for Mother's Day. Her desire is that her children will show her love all year round and not just on one day of the year.

This past Mother's Day was one I was not looking forward to. It was the fourth Mother's Day since we began trying to conceive, and it was by far the hardest. The first year I don't remember too much, so I suppose I was okay. That might have been the year that my kind husband brought me flowers in honor of the fact that I would one day be a mother. (He is such an amazing support to me!)

The second Mother's Day was a little more emotional. At that point I was serving as the coordinator for the baby dedications at our church, which we regularly held on Mother's Day. My Sunday morning was filled with oohing and aahing over babies dressed in their Sunday best, communicating with the families who came to the brunch, and helping the dedication portion of the church service run smoothly.

What was I thinking, coordinating baby dedications while I was unable to become pregnant? I was thinking that I love babies, and I'm going to serve and rejoice for others regardless of my personal status. That morning I stood back and thought about the families lined up across the front of the church to dedicate their infants to God. Since I personally knew many of the families, I realized that several of the couples up there had struggled to become pregnant. I was not alone. Miracle babies were all around, and it boosted my faith to know that if God could work a miracle for these couples, then He could do it for us. At that point friends knew we were trying to start a family, so I received some nice words of encouragement and even a thoughtful note or two.

The third Mother's Day I spent alone, since Mike was out of the country attending a wedding. I went to church that morning, where I fought back tears during the service, then I ran some errands and went to the gym. I remember going into a grocery store that had a salad bar, and in the mid-afternoon as I paid for my small salad the cashier said, "Happy Mother's Day if you have kids" or something like that. I resisted the urge to snap back, "If I had children, would I be here in my workout clothes buying a tiny little salad on Mother's Day?" I was definitely feeling sorry for myself.

Then the fourth Mother's Day approached. Although I felt okay most of the time, I wanted to escape from people I knew that day. Our current church is overflowing with young families and babies, and I didn't know if I could hold my emotions together that Sunday. When my husband coordinated a visit to his cousin's home in Pennsylvania that particular weekend, I was grateful. This cousin and his wife don't have children and I thought it would be ideal to spend Mother's Day with another childless couple.

That morning we attended a local church and heard a fabulous sermon about Mary, one of the most special mothers in history. Knowing that the ushers would be handing out flowers to all the moms at the main entrance, I slipped out a side door. Mike and I, along with his cousin and his wife, had an early lunch and visited a tourist site in the area.

Then Mike and I headed home – we had a several hour drive from Pittsburgh to Washington, D.C. Foolishly, and maybe desperately, I brought up the topic of adoption that day, as it had been weighing on my mind. When we travel, I talk with Mike almost nonstop.

It's a wonderful time to converse without too many interruptions, so it seemed fine to bring up a sensitive subject like adoption. But, I was feeling some PMS that day – and we didn't have any snacks in the car.

You know what happens when a woman is hungry and upset? She becomes hangry. (Hungry + angry = hangry, and hangry women say things that they shouldn't!) I soon realized that this was a bad combination: a hungry, hormonal woman, who wants children, talking about whether or not to adopt, on Mother's Day.

I tried to hold my emotions together in the beginning of the conversation, but we had decided that while we were in Pennsylvania we would stop to see the Flight 93 Memorial. Flight 93 was the airplane that was hijacked by terrorists on September 11, 2001, and from all the information that has been gathered, the passengers fought back. Realizing that the passengers would overpower them before they could follow through with their plan, the terrorists then crashed the plane into a Pennsylvania field instead of into the Capitol building in Washington, D.C. The memorial site was simple and the mood was quite somber. I fought back tears as I walked through the memorial, but unfortunately it turned on the waterworks.

I cried for the next hour or two of the drive. When we finally did walk into a restaurant at eight o'clock that night with my red swollen eyes and no children, I was grateful that the waitress didn't even try to wish us a Happy Mother's Day.

That day a good friend emailed me an article from EveryBitterThingIsSweet.com[1] that said as a woman trying to conceive for years, you have to put on a thick skin so as not to be offended or hurt all the time. Mother's Day, she said, is a fine time to shed that thick skin and get real before God.

Most of the time I might seem okay, and most of the time I am okay, yet deep down inside is a tremendous emptiness – a longing for children of my own that will only truly be fulfilled by children of my own.

One of the many blessings in my life right now is my job as a nanny for four little ones. Caring for a baby (now a toddler) all day and having a motherly role towards these little children certainly fills a void, but it's still not the same as having our own little ones.

I am healthy and able to have a happy life simply because of the covering God has placed over me. I cling to His grace, His comfort, and His promise. Still, there are times I break down, often monthly, and I cry myself to sleep in my husband's arms or fight tears at the news of yet another friend or family member having a baby. There are times when I take off my coat of armor and cry.

Psalm 30:5 shares a nugget of truth and wisdom, "Weeping may stay for the night, but rejoicing comes in the morning." Or as The Message translation says, "The nights of crying your eyes out give way to days of laughter."

When I look at the big picture, I know that even though our circumstances cause us to weep, God still brings us joy. I choose to hope for that day when God turns my weeping into laughter. Psalm 113 is a beautiful Psalm, and verse 9 paints the picture of a God who "settles the barren woman in her home as the happy mother of children." (1984 NIV) The description has many key points – this woman was once barren, now she is settled, in her home, she's happy, she's a mother, and she has children. I believe that God can do that.

Another struggle that I face is that I tend to be a worrier and a planner. Maybe there are women who go through life unconcerned about what's next, without worrying about the future, but I'm certainly not one of them. I like a plan for each and every day, and I thrive with a to-do list in hand. However, it only makes sense to plan what we can control, and much of life we can't. My children have certainly not come on schedule. If they had followed my plan, I would probably have a three-year-old and a one-year-old by now. Sometimes it's hard when I look at little ones who are around those same ages – I feel a stab of sadness, feeling like I'm missing out.

Holidays have often been difficult. We began trying for a baby early in the summer of 2010. I wondered if we would have a baby announcement for our families when we visited them later that same summer. When that didn't happen, I thought, *Well maybe we will be able to inform people that we're pregnant on our anniversary in November? Nope, well maybe Thanksgiving? Christmas? Maybe I'll find out that I'm pregnant on my birthday?* It's so easy to look ahead with wishful thinking: *If we can time it right, we can tell people that we're pregnant on Mother's Day.* Websites calculate due dates in an instant, leading me to speculate that if I get pregnant on this particular day then a baby would be due on a special day such as Mike's birthday. However, each passing birthday reminds me that we are getting older, and we are still childless. I'm learning that wishful thinking often leads to disappointment and that choosing to have a disciplined thought life decreases unnecessary disappointment and pain.

Month after month and holiday after holiday marched on. On many of those occasions I felt a pang of sadness, and sometimes I cried. Finally, after more than four years, I have mostly quit looking at the calendar, wondering when I'll become pregnant and dreaming up Pinterest-worthy baby announcements. Yes, I still hope and believe that the day will come, but maybe because my life is very full right now I'm obsessing less.

Many couples struggle to conceive, often for unknown reasons. According to resolve.org[2], one out of eight couples has a tough time either becoming pregnant or carrying a pregnancy to full term. Research attributes infertility in one-third of couples to the woman, one-third of the time to the man, and the other third is linked to both parties or unknown causes.

Since difficulty conceiving is a deeply personal topic, many people do not want to talk about it. Not only is the fertility struggle very personal, it's often emotionally painful, and it seems to a woman who is unable to become pregnant that most people cannot understand. Yet statistics show that more than ten percent of couples are facing a similar battle.

The fact is, we are not alone in this struggle, and furthermore there is a devil who really doesn't like us and doesn't want us to bring babies into this world. He wants us to be miserable throughout the process. He whispers lies into our heads such as "you're the only one going through this," or "it will never happen." I have found that by learning to focus on what God says instead of what the devil says or what my overly-emotional feelings say will completely shift the way I handle this struggle.

Fertility problems are so personal. Experiencing a lack of success in conceiving a baby involves disappointed hopes. Conversations about it can easily dig into a person's most personal matters: their health, their finances, and their sex life. Speaking of that intimate act, many couples trying to conceive for a long time admit that it strains their sexual relationship. When physical intimacy with your spouse is closely linked to attempting to conceive a baby, it can begin to feel more like a scientific process than an act of love. Although sex is an important part of a covenant marriage, and while it's where babies come from, if life or health hinder you from trying to conceive on just the right day, relax. Stay emotionally connected to your spouse, and know that with or without perfectly timed sex, God can do anything.

Struggling to conceive is very private. Talking to someone about one's fertility struggle is about as much fun as putting on that paper gown at the gynecologist's office and sticking two feet into the stirrups, exposing that most personal side to others.

In addition, the fertility challenge is a long slow process. If the average menstrual cycle is 28 days, then a woman only has 12–13 times each year in which she can conceive. We can "try" to get pregnant more than once within that time, but the fertile window surrounding ovulation is only a few days long. Other personal goals, such as running a 5K race in a certain time, could be attempted over and over again. Trying to get pregnant means that once a month we will get test results about whether or not you passed, and if we were unsuccessful, we wait two weeks before we can try again. Then we must wait two weeks for the results. It's a long wait, it's boring, and it's an emotional roller coaster.

Let's start with the beginning – at least this is how it goes in my head. I start my period. For me there is a lot of physical pain and a general feeling of misery for a couple of days. In past years I have missed days of school or work when on my period because at times the pain was so intense that I cannot function. Now, if I had tried to conceive that previous cycle, the pain and misery is compounded with deep disappointment and questioning God: *Will You ever answer my request for a child?*

Then as the period fades away, hope resurfaces. I'm sure hormonal shifts play into these emotions. After the pain is gone, I find fresh hope that maybe, just maybe, this will be the month that we conceive.

Soon ovulation comes, and as science has proven this is the time of the month when a woman feels the best overall. So not only do I feel good physically and emotionally, I feel good about myself, and I feel so much hope that it will work this time!

Post ovulation, my hormones shift and my hope sinks. In my case, I have pretty distinctive PMS: cramps, headaches, tender breasts, general sensations of not feeling so well. Historically, for the past twenty years, that means that my time of the month is just around the corner. In all my years of trying to conceive, so far these symptoms have just been PMS, not some new weird pregnancy symptom. Disappointment often hits me hard as my cycle starts.

The cycle begins again.

Thankfully, it's a cycle. Hope follows disappointment, then hope fades away as disappointment rises. I believe that one day disappointment will give way to a hope fulfilled.

Mike and I are doing all we can. We have both lost weight and have begun eating healthier. We keep an eye on my fertility charts to make sure we are trying to conceive at the most fertile time of the month. We pray together daily for a baby.

I've prayed out loud, "We just want a baby, Jesus!" To which Mike, with his dry sense of humor, interjects, "Actually, God, we don't want a baby Jesus, we just want a baby."

God certainly knows our desire for a child, and it feels like we have prayed from every imaginable perspective: asking God, rebuking the devil, repenting of my sins, asking God for healing, speaking life to my body, and asking many others to pray.

Whether our prayers are simple or exhaustive, we wait in expectancy for God to answer.

So many things can hinder a couple from even trying to get pregnant. For example, when one spouse is traveling or when both work long hours, it can be difficult to find the time for physical intimacy during the fertile days. Numerous health problems can interfere in the process. Although the reasons why a couple has difficulty conceiving are varied, the emotional struggle is similar.

I feel annoyed by well-meaning people who say things like, "Just relax and before you know it you'll be pregnant!" In our years of wanting a baby, there have been relaxed months and not-so-relaxed months, times when I was fully distracted by some other life event, and times when I was overly focused on what day of my cycle it happened to be. Nothing has worked so far.

I've learned that I can't completely take charge of my fertility. I'm not in control of when my babies come. Do I like it? No. Have I come to grips with it? Mostly. Do I believe God is doing something through it? Yes.

A child that I nanny went through a phase of responding to my simple instructions (such as "put on your shoes") with flailing arms and wailing, "Why are you doing this to me!?" I would do my best to not laugh outright at the ridiculousness of the child's response, for I knew what we needed to accomplish at that time.

Likewise, I could turn to God and raise my fist and ask, "Why God? Why are You being so mean to me by not giving me a baby?"

The fact is, He's not mean. He's good. He knows what He's doing, because He sees the big picture.

Inside my head any time I'm praying or worshipping God, I'm often being reminded by God that He is good, or I'm reminding myself that He is good. I'm crying out to Him to provide children to us when His time is right, in the way that He wants. Things have certainly not gone according to my plan, so I know that His plan will be the way that it will be, and I choose to trust His character, believing that He is good.

Throughout the Bible we read that His character is good. The Psalms repeat it many times:

> "Taste and see that the Lord is good; blessed is the one who takes refuge in Him." Psalm 34:8

> "For the Lord is good and His love endures forever; His faithfulness continues through all generations." Psalm 100:5

> "Give thanks to the Lord, for He is good; His love endures forever." Psalm 107:1

Even though His Word says that He's good, sometimes circumstances leave us wondering.

The first time I seriously questioned the goodness of God was in 2004 when I was serving on a mission trip with the medical mission agency I worked for at the time. We were in Suriname, South America, holding medical clinics in prisons.

While any prison is a tough place to visit, juvenile detention centers in a third-world country are worse.

After our team wrapped up our medical clinic in the juvenile detention center one afternoon, we were given a tour of the cells where these boys lived. Entering a courtyard through a huge metal door, I looked up to see barbed wire crisscrossed above the entire courtyard, like a ceiling, allowing no escape. It felt like a giant cage.

Beyond the courtyard were an office and cells. This facility was designed to be a temporary holding place for teens awaiting court hearings.

Boys, teenagers, and some not quite even teenagers were locked into tiny bare cells with nothing but a bunk bed, a five-gallon bucket that could be used as a toilet, and another prisoner. Some were there for drug offenses or more serious crimes, and some were there for simple theft such as stealing bread in order to survive. I cannot fathom a facility like this existing in the United States.

This was not a place for teenage boys to straighten out their lives; it seemed more like a cage for animals. My heart broke as I stood in that concrete walkway and looked around. At that time, I worked closely with the youth group at my church, and I couldn't imagine the young boys I knew surviving in such a place. My brother was a teenager then, and one of the boys reminded me very much of him. I couldn't imagine my brother being locked up in such a place.

As I stood outside the bars with my teammates, the boys sang a song in English that they had learned from a pastor who visited them. The chorus resonated off the walls and stayed in my mind for years to come:

> God is a good God, yes He is
> God is a good God, yes He is
> He picks me up and turns me 'round
> He sets my feet on higher ground.

I remember in that moment asking myself, *How could anyone in those circumstances joyfully sing that God is good? If I were confined to one of those cells, I don't know that I would be singing about God's goodness.* Yet those boys seemed to deeply understand that God is good.

Later that day I stood in the shower washing away the grime and the stress of the day, and as I savored my rare moment of solitude on a mission trip, my heart cried out to God: *How? How can they say that You are good when they're living like that?*

In one of the most vivid instances of God speaking to my heart, I heard Him say, "Betsy, don't doubt that I am good."

Since then I have certainly wondered about God's goodness. I have questioned and even doubted. Still one of the most distinct things that I have ever heard God say to me personally is that He is GOOD. One of the key things is that I have learned to separate God's character from the circumstances around me. Even when things look worse than I could imagine, He is still good.

As His timing would have it, I returned home from that week away to face hardships in my circle of friends, including broken marriages and deaths. Situations like these tempted me to accuse God of not being good, however, His whisper to me on that mission trip resonated in my heart.

That same year I began working at the local 911 dispatching center where I spent several years hearing the details of rapes, murders, unpleasant deaths, and devastating house fires. Many of these situations that I dealt with as a 911 dispatcher sent me home in tears, again wondering how God could be good.

However, He said that He is good, both in the Bible and by speaking directly to my heart. So I choose to believe it.

Now, more than a decade later, I have not forgotten the place where God showed me that He is good despite the circumstances. Today I can look at my greatest dream not happening yet and know that God is good and He is loving. So now when I find myself feeling down I know to ask myself if I am focusing on the circumstances or on God?

Several years ago a couple from our church at the time lost their six-month-old baby girl to SIDS. This couple, Jon and Kelley Owens, were very visible in our church since Jon was the worship pastor. Baby Aria went to Heaven on a Wednesday evening while I was at church teaching the children's program. In fact, I remember the exact place I was standing when I heard that she had stopped breathing during her nap at home and had been rushed to the hospital where she was pronounced dead.

Although I never held that baby, I remember when her mom was pregnant with her. I remember the play-by-play updates on Facebook when Kelley went into labor, I remember Aria's red hair, and I remember the day that she was dedicated to the Lord at our church. Her six months on earth left an impression on many.

Her sudden death impacted me, but what has impacted me even more is that Jon and Kelley continue to live with grace and trust that God is still good. Jon had just introduced a song to our church weeks before, and he sang it again at his daughter's memorial service.

Hope's Anthem
written by William Matthews & Christa Black Gifford [3]

> He's awakening the hope in me
> By calling forth my destiny
> He's breathing life into my soul
> I will thirst for Him, and Him alone
> He has come like the rain
> That showers on the barren plain
> So my heart and tongue confess
> Jesus Christ, the hope of man
>
> My hope is in You, God
> I am steadfast, I will not be moved
> I'm anchored, never shaken
> All my hope is in You

God showers hope on barren plains; He also showers hope into saddened hearts and barren wombs. "My hope is in you, God, I am steadfast, I will not be moved." Those words give me goose bumps every time I read them. When that song runs through my head, or if I sing it as I go about my day, my heart says "yes!"

If that grieving daddy could stand before our congregation and sing that his hope is in God, then I can walk through my sorrow with hope as well. They grieve the loss of their baby, which is a pain I don't want to imagine. I grieve a lack of babies, which is also painful.

Since losing Aria, Jon and Kelley have pressed forward in life. While writing this book, I watched via the internet as they sang and spoke during a worship service.

Kelley's declaration of truth as written in the "Prologue to the Fall"[4] still resonates in my heart:

> He is, after all, the Lord of all,
> both sorrow and joy,
> in the rise and the fall.
> And our falling in worship
> defines this our trust:

He is always good,
and we are always loved.
He is always good,
and we are always loved.

When we have faith that God is always good and that He always loves us, then there is always hope. I want to be like the woman described in Proverbs 31:25: "She is clothed with strength and dignity; she can laugh at the days to come." No matter what the past, present, or future hold, I will choose to believe that God is good and therefore I can stand steadfast in Him.

Chapter 7 – I'm Not Alone

By yourself you're unprotected.
With a friend you can face the worst...
Ecclesiastes 4:12 (The Message)

When we first began trying to conceive and the months passed without a positive pregnancy test, I would look around at the women in my social circles and complain to Mike that we were the only couple who couldn't get pregnant. I later realized that many women fight this battle silently. One by one I found others who were also having difficulty conceiving. I keep meeting women who want to have a baby, but it just isn't happening. Now I know that I am not alone.

One day I searched for infertility books at my local library, and I came across the book *Finding Grace* by Donna VanLiere[1]. This story told of her years attempting to conceive. Like me, Donna is a Christian, and like me, she clung to the Scripture that says God can put the barren mother in her home as the happy mother of children. Throughout her story, she came to realize that it was unlikely that she would give birth to children, and she and her husband were both in favor of pursuing adoption at that point. She is now the happy mother of three children through adoption and she has written some powerful fiction books about grace, family, and adoption.

Although Mike and I have been trying to get pregnant for over four years, I still believe that God will faithfully answer our prayers for a child in my womb. If He answers differently, such as by giving me children by adoption, then I will continue to trust and believe that He is good and He is in charge. Later in the book, I will delve deeper into my thoughts about adoption as a possible solution for childless couples.

I heard a beautiful adoption announcement that sent my heart soaring. Lynette Lewis is married to Ron Lewis, pastor of the church where Mike and I first met. When she married him, she became a stepmother to four sons, although she longed for babies of her own. Over the years she shared freely that she desired to have a baby. Mike and I prayed often that she would have children, and we hoped that He would fulfill her dream.

Then God, who loves to fulfill the desires of our hearts, gave Lynette beautiful twin newborn girls through adoption when she was 51 years old. Although those babies were not of her own womb, they were a supernatural gift from a God who answers the cries of our hearts.

She is not the only woman who has been surprised by God with babies later in life. The Patriarchs of our Christian faith are Abraham, Isaac, and Jacob. Did you know that each of them had a long wait for babies to come?

Hebrews 12:1 describes a great cloud of witnesses – those who lived before we did, who were full of faith in God. I'm fascinated by these women who dreamed of being mothers, only to be answered by God much later than they anticipated. I imagine these women in Heaven are cheering me on. "*Betsy, four years has been hard, but I waited forty. You can do it.*"

Sarah

Sarah is a logical place to start, as she is most famously known for having her first baby late in life. I distinctly remember a couple of winters ago when I walked into a Bible Study group for the first time. The lesson was about Abraham and Sarah conceiving their miracle baby Isaac. One key point that the speaker made was that "All of God's promises are Yea and Amen." The speaker, originally from Kenya, had a lovely British accent.

As she spoke the words "Yea and Amen" she pronounced "Yea" as I would say "Yay" in my American accent. She was saying that God's promises are Yes and Amen, as the Scripture states in 2 Corinthians 1:20, but I heard a "Yay" deep in my spirit – knowing that when God's promises come to pass, we can't help but to respond with a "Yay!" So when I think of that verse, I hear in my mind that God's promises are, "Yes! Yay! And Amen!"

"Yays!" are shouted when miracle babies come to be. I believe that there are more miracle babies yet to be conceived – in us and in many other couples. Many more "Yays!" will one day be heard.

In that hormonal crash when I'm PMSing and crying to Mike, "Will we ever get pregnant?" or when we feel like no hope is left, there is hope. Even if we were to blatantly doubt God or laugh in the face of His promises, there is still hope, as Sarah has demonstrated.

Sarah, Abraham's wife, is mentioned in Hebrews 11, the chapter commonly known as the "Hall of Faith" in the Bible. The writer of Hebrews says in verse 11, "And by faith even Sarah, who was past childbearing age, was enabled to bear children because she considered Him faithful who had made the promise." Although that Scripture is concise and beautiful, focusing on Sarah's faith in God's promise, she didn't demonstrate her faith at all times.

Long after Sarah's childbearing years were over, God came to Abraham (who was named Abram at that point, but I'll call him Abraham to keep it simple) and told him not to be afraid for God is his shield and reward (Genesis 15). God told Abraham that he would have a son who is his own flesh and blood, and that he would have as many offspring as the stars in the sky. Since it seemed that Sarah (Sarai before her name change) would not bear children, this couple took matters into their own hands and went with the sensible fertility option in their time: Sarah gave Abraham her handmaiden so he could have a baby with her. Abraham and Hagar together had Ishmael, who was not the son that God promised. So God came back later and visited Abraham again.

Abraham was 86 when Ishmael was born. The Bible records his next encounter with God when he was 99. Again God promised

Abraham that he and Sarah would have a child together. If they didn't think Sarah was too old 14 years before that point, they certainly would have thought it was impossible then! Before Sarah's famous laugh, as recorded in Genesis 17:17, Abraham fell on his face before God chuckling and asked himself, "Will a son be born to a man a hundred years old? Will Sarah bear a child at the age of ninety?" (I might have laughed too: my grandmothers are 90-ish and I cannot fathom either of them having a baby now!) Later, the angels of the Lord came and told Abraham, "I will surely return to you about this time next year, and Sarah your wife will have a son." That's when Sarah laughed, but nonetheless, a year later Isaac was born!

God wasn't rendered powerless by her age. A friend in her forties who desires babies of her own once shared with me that even though it's upsetting to get a monthly period, it's actually more devastating when her period does not come one month, indicating that menopause is around the corner. Obviously, hope diminishes when a woman's body begins menopause. Yet God is greater.

Bill Johnson, pastor of Bethel Church in Redding, CA, spoke about Sarah in his Mother's Day message in 2014 (titled "Birthing the Impossible"[2]). He points out that in Genesis, Sarah laughed at God's word about giving birth, and then she lied about it, denying it. Yet in the New Testament, Sarah is noted as a woman of faith. Bill Johnson says that, "Sarah received strength when she considered Him faithful... Her role was to think about His faithfulness."

Regardless of her attempt to take matters into her own hands by having her husband sleep with her servant to conceive his first son, Sarah goes down in history for having faith that God could do it. God sees us with His eyes of love. In spite of Sarah's mistakes and poor responses, somehow she ultimately believed God and that affected how God saw her.

As I write today, I am 34, Mike is 46. When we got married, I was 28 and Mike was 40. I often feel like we (especially Mike) will be much older parents than "everybody else." It's not that our bodies can't conceive at these ages – I just don't want to be older parents than my peers. But it's out of my control.

So I read about these heroes in the Bible.

Are we too old to have children? Not from God's perspective, and His outlook defines mine. Sure, my husband will be an older dad than most, but at least he won't be as old as Abraham!

Just the other day Mike and I were participating in a worship event. He was reading some verses in Psalms while I sang and played the guitar, and as he read Psalm 92 aloud we looked at each other and laughed. Verses 14–15 spoke to us:

> They will still bear fruit in old age,
> they will stay fresh and green,
> proclaiming, "The LORD is upright;
> He is my Rock, and there is no wickedness in Him."

Abraham

Romans 4:18–21 says:

> Against all hope,
> Abraham in hope believed
> and so became the father of many nations,
> just as it had been said to him,
> "So shall your offspring be."
>
> Without weakening in his faith,
> he faced the fact that his body was as good as dead –
> since he was about a hundred years old –
> and that Sarah's womb was also dead.
>
> Yet he did not waver through unbelief
> regarding the promise of God,
> but was strengthened in his faith
> and gave glory to God,
> being fully persuaded that God
> had power to do what He had promised.

This Scripture describes it well, starting with "against all hope." Abraham believed God when He said that they would have a child, even though it did not seem realistic in the natural sense. Against all logic and reason, Abraham still had a glimmer of hope. His body didn't seem like it was up to the job of procreating. His wife's reproductive system had shut down.

Yet God.

God spoke. God promised offspring. Abraham didn't waver – he was strengthened in his faith and he gave glory to God, knowing without a doubt that God was able to do what He had promised.

And He did.

Rebekah

Often the Bible refers to "the God of Abraham, Isaac, and Jacob." Those three guys were vital to God's story of His people; they are the patriarchs of our faith and each one had a wife who struggled to become pregnant. Isaac, Jacob, Joseph, and Benjamin were children who were born after years of prayers – they were divinely appointed by God. Not that children who are conceived right away can't be key figures in God's kingdom, but it seems to me that there is something remarkable about those children in the Bible who are asked of God for a very long time. I wonder if asking God for children for years and years might just mean that God is using those prayers to shape a mighty man or woman for His kingdom. God is also shaping us as the adults who will parent these children.

Isaac, the son of God's promise to Abraham, was born when his parents were 90 and 100. The story of how he met his wife Rebekah is one of a divine appointment. Abraham sent his servant back to their homeland to find a wife for Isaac, assuring him that God would send His angel ahead of the servant so that he could find a wife for Isaac. So the servant set out on his mission with ten camels.

When he approached the town, the servant brought his camels to a well and asked God for a specific sign – that the woman God intended to be Isaac's wife would be the one that when he approached wouldn't just offer him a drink, but would also water his camels.

Genesis 24:15–16 points out that "Before he had finished praying, Rebekah came out with her jar on her shoulder… The woman was very beautiful, a virgin…"

He asked her for a drink, and she shared water with him, then just as he had asked God, the woman offered to draw well water for the camels. Rebekah demonstrated a great attitude, kindness, and the willingness to serve. It is interesting to me that God answered the servant's prayer so quickly. Because He's God, He sometimes answers prayers by immediately granting the request, and other times He takes much longer.

The servant and Rebekah's father went through the arrangement of the marriage, then he brought her home to Isaac. Genesis 24:67 says that Isaac brought her into his tent and married her. "So she became his wife, and he loved her."

Sounds like a perfect little love story: man seeks wife, matchmaker sent, prayers prayed, woman willing, man loves woman, they marry.

If I were writing this story, they would have many children, the first being born about nine months after they wed.

But God likes authoring our love stories – and our parenting stories.

Their fertility quest is summed up concisely. Genesis 25:21 says, "Isaac prayed to the Lord on behalf of his wife, because she was childless. The Lord answered his prayer, and his wife Rebekah became pregnant."

One verse. Not a long story. Reading that verse just on the surface it seems like, "Oh how nice, virgins married and after a couple of months, when a baby didn't come along, Isaac said a prayer and BOOM, Rebekah was pregnant."

Nope, that verse covers decades of time. Isaac was 40 when they married. Verse 26 of that chapter states that "Isaac was sixty years old when Rebekah gave birth."

Twenty years, or probably nineteen, went by from the time they married until they conceived. The birth control pill or other methods of contraception were not holding them back. I expect that they were naturally trying to conceive: no contraception, no fertility treatments. God's promise for many descendants to Abraham applied to his son Isaac as well, and I imagine that Isaac knew that. Kids were supposed to be part of the package deal, right God? Yet God's ways are higher, His reasoning is different than ours.

Isaac and Rebekah experienced *years* of waiting. Wondering. Trying. Praying. They waited twenty years from the time they married until the time she gave birth, and four is feeling awfully long to me.

But God answers prayers. And sometimes, just because He can, He gives a double portion unexpectedly. Rebekah found out "when the time came for her to give birth, there were twin boys in her womb." (Genesis 25:24)

As one who has thought endlessly about ovulation and menstrual cycles, I wonder what held Rebekah's body back from conception, other than God's timing? Why did He allow twenty years between marriage and the birth of her twins? And how did a woman who presumably had never become pregnant suddenly produce two eggs – fraternal twins? I do not know the answer to all my speculative questions, other than "it's God."

Why did God have Rebekah wait twenty years? I do not know. I do know, however, that God's timing is right, despite our lack of understanding. Perhaps He included the story of her long wait to encourage women struggling to conceive today.

Rachel

A long wait for children happened again in the next generation. After Rebekah gave birth to her twins, Jacob and Esau, they had some drama-filled sibling rivalry, although God ultimately worked things out according to His plan. Jacob's sons became the twelve tribes of Israel, and through the tribe of Judah came the Lion of Judah, Jesus.

Jacob wanted to marry a beautiful young lady named Rachel. She was from the right family line, and she had certainly caught his eye. Genesis 29:14–30 tells a story that I find interesting. To make a long story short, Jacob asked Laban if he could marry his daughter Rachel. Laban agreed that after Jacob worked for him for seven years then he could marry his daughter. Those years passed and the wedding came – and Laban tricked Jacob by marrying him to his oldest daughter, who the Bible describes as having weak eyes, and we presume that she was not as desirable as her younger sister. Jacob confronted his father-in-law who agreed to let him marry Rachel the next week, as long as he promised to work for him for another seven years. That is how Jacob came to be married to two sisters: Leah and Rachel.

Considering that Jacob had previously done his share of tricking family members, he might have gotten what he deserved. Yet he also worked for fourteen years to earn these two wives, one whom he wanted and the other that he was tricked into marrying.

It turned out that Rachel was unable to conceive, and she was the much-loved wife, so we can presume that a lack of sex life was not the issue, right?

For reasons I don't fully understand, Genesis 29:31 says, "When the Lord saw that Leah was not loved, He enabled her to conceive, but Rachel remained childless." Leah went on to have several children. However, Rachel was not getting pregnant even though she was the favored wife. She tried the same fertility method that her husband's grandparents had tried – she gave her husband a handmaiden to have some babies for her. (This was the surrogate mothering of that day.) Leah also had some more babies in the meantime, both through her handmaiden and through her own body.

In her jealousy and desperation, Rachel said to her husband, "Give me children, or I'll die!" Have you ever felt like that?

Genesis 30:22–24 says, "Then God remembered Rachel; He listened to her and enabled her to conceive. She became pregnant and gave birth to a son and said, 'God has taken away my disgrace.' She named him Joseph, and said, 'May the Lord add to me another son.'"

God then added another son to Rachel, whose name was Benjamin. He was the final son of the twelve.

If you look closely at Joseph's life you'll see that he was used to save the people of Israel and the surrounding areas from dying from a famine. Could it be that the Lord delayed his birth so that he would be able to lead a nation at just the right time?

God knew the right times for each one of Jacob's children to be born. Could it be that God has a plan for my children that is bigger than my imagination? And that His timing is perfect?

This trio of mother-in-laws and daughter-in-laws Sarah, Rebekah, and Rachel, are not the only three women in Scripture who had difficulty bearing children. I will share more stories as we continue.

We are not alone in this struggle to conceive.

God is a God who gives and takes away, and also sometimes He doesn't give. We often do not immediately understand why, and we frequently do not like it. But ultimately we have to believe that there is a purpose for it and that God has a rhyme and reason for what is happening. In the long run, life is easier when we choose to trust Him.

In our culture, we grieve when someone loses a child, and we rejoice when a child is born. But what about the woman and her husband who desperately want a child of their own yet do not have one? How do we as a community respond? Do we grieve? Do we even know that this couple is going through this silent struggle?

I'm not the only woman who several years ago thought that she'd have a baby by the spring. I'm not the only one staring ahead at her thirty-fifth or fortieth birthday, knowing that the doctor will check my eggs to see if they seem to be too old.

I think it's wonderful for couples to get married and have children right away, despite the common philosophy that "it's good to have some years to yourself." In fact, I would have been willing to start a family, or at least to begin trying, a few months into our marriage. However, Mike felt that it would be better to wait longer than a few months. Being newly married and trying to figure out how to get along with my new husband, it seemed wise to agree with him. So in our second year of marriage, he gave the green light and we began trying to conceive. Seasons of disappointment and discouragement, contrasted with deepening hope and faith have marked the years since we began trying to start our family.

It seemed that nearly all of my friends and family members had gotten pregnant almost immediately after stopping birth control (and those who didn't go the route of birth control managed to get pregnant on their honeymoon). Several friends have even managed to conceive before actually trying to, so I expected to become pregnant quickly.

In our church at the time, having babies seemed to be the standard for married women in their twenties and thirties. Pregnant bellies were everywhere, along with babies strapped onto a parent's chest in some sort of baby carrier, strollers clogging the aisles, and toddlers climbing up and down the steps. Our church nursery was overwhelmingly full. I remember a Sunday when I was teaching the two-year-olds and we had twenty-six of them in our class that day. I felt very out of place with my empty arms. Yet as I began to find other women in my church who weren't able to have babies quite so easily, I realized that I was not alone.

I'm more than not alone – I'm finding out that I am surrounded by others who are currently in this struggle. I also draw strength from those women mentioned in the Bible who successfully fought this battle long ago. I'm constantly reminded that God is good, He is faithful, and He is in control. I've been able to walk through this season with a supernatural grace; I've grown in my faith.

As I look around and see that I'm not in this battle by myself, I also gain more clarity that the devil, our greatest enemy, wants each of us in similar situations to feel isolated. However, he lies. In a later chapter I'll dig further into our great need to focus on the truths that God speaks to us.

In our journey of trying to start a family, I have learned that it's easier to tell people how it's going – at least to some degree. On the medical side of things, I have shared certain information with close friends or family, but I don't want people getting their hopes up that maybe this next procedure or medication will solve everything. Early on I learned to not tell anyone other than Mike on the occasions when I thought I might be pregnant, since following up with disappointing news was tough.

One reason I do not keep secret the fact that we're actively trying to start a family is because as strongly as I desire children, I don't want a single person to assume that I don't want kids. So I'm not shy to talk about the fact that we want to have a baby, and we freely tell people that we've been trying for several years to get pregnant. I find that this generates encouragement, prayers, and only the occasional unhelpful comments. Despite the words that annoy me, the prayers are worth it. The support is worth it.

I realize that I'm surrounded by a crowd of people, many who care, and I'm surrounded by some who have walked this road and understand. I feel like some bystanders in my life are just gawking at me, judging me, or thinking I should handle my circumstances differently. Some offer encouragement although their very fertile bodies hinder them from truly understanding the difficulty of what I'm going through.

I have found that I connect on a deeper level with those who are walking this same road, whether they're unable to get pregnant for the first time, or they miscarry when they do conceive, or they have already had children but can't get pregnant again. My heart goes out to other women who are trying without success. I also hurt for the women who desperately want to be wives and mothers, but remain unmarried. I was in that position for a season – just wanting to be a wife and then a mom – and it seemed impossible.

Friends, family, and social media connections continually encourage me. I am strengthened as I remember the women of faith in the Bible who have walked this road before. Hebrews 12:1–3 refers to those who have gone before us as a great cloud of witnesses who are now surrounding us. As I look around here on earth, I see a great crowd of witnesses cheering me on as I pursue my dream of becoming a mother.

Chapter 8 – Thoughts and Words

For though we walk in the flesh,
we do not war according to the flesh.
For the weapons of our warfare are not carnal
but mighty in God for pulling down strongholds,
casting down arguments and every high thing
that exalts itself against the knowledge of God,
bringing every thought into captivity
to the obedience of Christ.
2 Corinthians 10:3–5 (NKJV)

I do not like the word infertility. Although it's a term I use frequently since I'm writing a book on the topic, I prefer to not use it in describing myself. One thing I'm learning over the years is that words hold power, and words begin with a thought. 2 Corinthians 10:5 tells us to take every thought captive and make it obey Christ. About a year into this trying to conceive journey, I became aware of some thoughts that were negatively impacting me.

The spring after we began trying to start our family, Mike and I attended a week of ministry at the Restoring the Foundations (RTF)[1] headquarters in Hendersonville, North Carolina, a program headed by Chester and Betsy Kylstra. This was a life-changing week for us as God dealt with issues deep within us.

In a nutshell, I would describe this week as a combination of receiving counseling and prayer. We dedicated that week to dealing with baggage in our hearts, minds, and souls – wanting to get rid of harmful things that we might not even have been aware of. After spending a week with trained counselors, we walked away transformed. In hindsight, that week at RTF was a good turning point in our marriage, which certainly hadn't been bad before, but was even better after. It was a turning point individually as each of us overcame things that had held us back from God.

Although I had been a Christian since childhood, was determined to live a godly life, knew the Bible fairly well, and considered myself to be a pretty good person, I still discovered thoughts rooted deep inside of my heart that were actually lies. These lies were about God, about myself, and about others.

The counselors at RTF called these thoughts that contradict God's truths "ungodly beliefs." As I met and shared with this couple throughout the week, they wrote down the ungodly beliefs that they picked up on in my life (even if I wasn't aware of them). Then we spent one morning together where I repented to God for believing things contrary to the truth. With their help, I wrote out some new godly beliefs based on Scripture which they suggested that I meditate upon for the next few weeks. The purpose for meditating on these statements was to retrain my thinking so that I could walk in truth. Those statements are within easy reach to this day so that I can remind myself of what God says about me.

Intentionally shifting my thoughts to more truthful and godly thinking changed my heart. The heart change improved my emotions and I became more emotionally stable. Grasping more godly beliefs changed my view of God, which has allowed me to face trials with a newfound faith and hope.

As the Kylstras teach, our beliefs lead to our thoughts, our thoughts lead to our attitudes, our attitudes lead to our actions, our actions lead to our habits, our habits lead to our character, and our character leads to our destiny. It is vitally important that we understand and put this principle into practice.

The ministry time helped me to identify eight specific ungodly beliefs that I had fallen prey to, and although all of them tied into the fertility struggle, I will focus on two of these statements:

"I am not sure that God wants to give me good things so therefore I can't trust Him with my hopes and dreams of being a mother."

"God wants to bless everyone except for me."

I know for a fact that I felt this way before I met Mike: I felt like God liked my friends more than me, therefore He gave them godly spouses but withheld that gift from me! This incorrect perspective of God reappeared when I was not able to become pregnant. Doesn't Psalm 127:3 say that children are a blessing from the Lord? Well, I assumed that for some reason God didn't want to bless me, therefore He must not love me, or I must have done something wrong. However, I came to see that the source behind my thoughts was the devil, who is our enemy.

Sally M. Jones, in her book *Longing Heart; Empty Arms*[2], describes this scenario well, as one of her characters tells of how she and a friend "had talked recently about how Satan tried to put thoughts in their minds. They were always negative, against God, something to beat themselves up with, or something similar. They had both come to the conclusion that they really had to be on their guard against things like that and fight against it."

The Bible says that we should be transformed by the renewing of our minds (Romans 12:2). At RTF, I renounced the ungodly belief that God doesn't love me very much so He withholds gifts. Then I began to reprogram my thinking with God's Biblical truths. I began to focus on Psalm 103:5, declaring that God satisfies my desires with good things. I remembered that Psalm 37:4 says that He will give us the desires of our hearts. I began to believe and meditate on the fact that God is for me, not against me (Romans 8:31). I am also strengthened when I listen to and sing songs that reinforce that truth. It was around this time that I began to be encouraged by the beautiful imagery in Psalm 113:9 that describes a God who makes the barren woman a happy mother of children.

Month by month and year by year as I wrestle with this fertility challenge, I continue to discover ungodly beliefs in my heart. Just the other day, even as I was knee-deep in writing this chapter, we shared our situation with a woman from our church. Mike told her our ages then I attempted a joke by saying, "I'm getting older every day!" The woman, Mike, and I all realized immediately that those words were not life-giving – at 34 I'm definitely not too old to conceive. I repented to the Lord and am making intentional efforts to choose my thoughts and words carefully and not to see our ages as hindrances to conception.

In light of that, I have taken deeply to heart the truth that God is for me. And the fact is, the devil is against us. Recently I was reading a book called *A Million Little Ways: Uncover the Art You Were Made to Live* by Emily P. Freeman[3]. She said, "I can't imagine anything more dangerous to the enemy of our hearts than people who know who they are."

Knowing who we are as women loved by God and knowing that our calling to motherhood is unquestionable will only make us stronger and more capable of walking out our destiny.

However, our thoughts are the foundation of our words, and just as I try to speak words that are life-giving, I also need to take my thoughts captive. 2 Corinthians 10:5 tells us to take every thought captive and make it obey Christ. This means that we should examine our thoughts to see where they have come from: are they simply from our own minds, or are they thoughts from God, or perhaps even from the enemy? If we know that the thought is from the enemy, we need to get it out of our minds and replace it with God's truth. If we're not sure where the thought is from or how valid it is, we should compare it to God's character and His Word – if it's not in agreement with God, then we need to take it captive and it needs to go. Ideally, this process should happen regularly in our minds, becoming part of how we think. As our minds become filled with true thoughts about God, those true thoughts can begin to come out of our mouths as life-giving words.

Before I met Mike, I was familiar with the idea of how the words we speak affect our lives, but I didn't really understand their power as well as I do now. The Bible says that there is life and death in the power of the tongue (Proverbs 18:21). We can choose to speak words that bless or words that curse, and James 3:1–12 makes it clear that both kind words and damaging things should not come from the same mouth.

"For the mouth speaks what the heart is full of," says Jesus in Luke 6:45. The thoughts and feelings inside of our hearts overflow out of our mouths, and the words spoken are powerful. Therefore, we must be careful with our thoughts and with our words. The words we say, even careless or seemingly trivial ones, have power to affect our lives, circumstances, bodies, and futures.

In my first few years with Mike, as we dated, were engaged, and were newlyweds, we had a number of conflicts regarding words. I would get mad and say bad things. He would be mad that I would say such things. I would be upset because he was mad, and then he would get mad because I was upset, at which point, whatever had triggered this cycle of events would be forgotten. But emotional words, spoken carelessly, certainly didn't help anything.

The principle of not speaking destructive words was something I was familiar with, but I found it to be surprisingly difficult to apply when I was upset, tired, angry, or emotional due to my ever-fluctuating hormones.

After months, years, or decades of trying to conceive, it's understandable to feel disappointed, angry, and generally unhappy every time a period comes. There are times in my cycle when I naturally feel more upbeat and hopeful, and speaking words of life over my circumstances is much easier.

Although it's really hard to speak life-giving words (rather than damaging ones) in the midst of disappointment and pain, words are powerful and it would be beneficial for us to do so. I admit that it is still a challenge for me to always put this into practice.

Infertility is a word that we have intentionally been very careful not to proclaim over our lives. Although we have not had babies yet, we refuse to call ourselves infertile.

Although I am a woman who doesn't have children, my identity is not found there. Truthfully, I relate very comfortably to moms because that's who I identify with.

Recently I joined a couple of infertility groups on Facebook, and from reading those posts, it seems that some people are completely focused on not being able to conceive. I definitely understand the need for support when facing a challenge, however it's very important to think about whether the focus is on the *difficulty* or the focus is on the *goal*. There is a big difference between meditating on the current reality, such as: "I am infertile" or on what God sees: "He designed me to mother children."

The words we say about ourselves absolutely affect the way that we see ourselves. That is one of the reasons why the tongue is so powerful.

The devil truly wants to make us miserable – or even more than that, John 10:10 says that the devil comes to steal, kill, and destroy. James 4:7 says, "Resist the devil, and he will flee from you." One way to resist the devil is to simply tell him to go away. Speaking God's truth is another way to overcome the enemy, as Jesus demonstrated when He was tested by the devil in the wilderness (Matthew 4:1–11).

Practically, we can resist the devil by speaking God's truth into our circumstances as my friend Mandy did. She spoke life to her womb and thanked God in advance for what she believed that He would do. Eventually she gave birth to a healthy baby girl. As a negative example of the power of speaking words to oneself, in my past I have spent months or years telling myself that I was overweight, or that I felt chubby. Sure enough, I put on some extra pounds during those years.

What we meditate on is also very influential in our lives. For example, about a year ago I began running for exercise, and as a result I began to think of myself as a runner. Shifting my focus from who I thought I was to who I could become allowed me to change for the better. More often than not these days I see myself as somewhat fit instead of as overweight.

Nearly every morning I ask the children that I nanny what kind of day they would like to have. Every day, despite their moods and feelings, these little ones tell me that they want to have a good day.

Speaking those words out loud helps to set the tone for the day ahead.

The words I say affect my identity as well as my destiny. Words and thoughts influence each other, and these can affect my relationship with God. The way that I see God most definitely affects how I handle this season of trying to start a family.

Although our circumstances may not change instantly, if we come to God sincerely asking Him to give us His perspective, that will change our thoughts, and consequently, how we view our circumstances will improve.

This is one of the most important reasons why I have held on to hope throughout our years of trying to conceive – my mind and heart have become more aligned with God's. Therefore I know that He is good, that His timing is right, and I am excited that He has allowed this past year to be one of the best in my life, despite the fact that one of my greatest dreams is yet unfulfilled.

Chapter 9 – Great Cloud of Witnesses

Therefore, since we are surrounded
by such a great cloud of witnesses,
let us throw off everything that hinders
and the sin that so easily entangles,
and let us run with perseverance
the race marked out for us.
Let us fix our eyes on Jesus,
the author and perfecter of our faith...
Hebrews 12:1–2 (1984 NIV)

Have you ever noticed that God's first appearance in the New Testament was to tell a childless elderly couple that they were going to become parents?

Did you know that all of the women mentioned in Jesus' genealogy were the moms of miracle babies?

Have you ever realized that Jesus Himself had something to say to a woman who had spent all of her money on doctors only to still have a bleeding problem?

Earlier I described the trio of women in the Bible who struggled to conceive: Sarah, Rebekah, and Rachel. They are not the only three women in Scripture who had difficulty bearing children. Many of the women we read about faced this challenge for decades, eventually having babies when it seemed completely impossible, in an age when medical assistance and modern resources did not exist. Here are more people in the great cloud of witnesses cheering us on from Heaven!

Elizabeth

Elizabeth and her husband Zechariah were an elderly couple introduced at the beginning of the New Testament. Luke 1:6–7 says "Both of them were righteous in the sight of God, observing all the Lord's commands and decrees blamelessly. But they were childless because Elizabeth was not able to conceive, and they were both very old."

One day it was Zechariah's turn to perform his priestly duties in the temple. He went in, and an angel of the Lord appeared and said in Luke 1:13–17:

> Do not be afraid, Zechariah; your prayer has been heard. Your wife Elizabeth will bear you a son, and you are to call him John. He will be a joy and delight to you, and many will rejoice because of his birth, for he will be great in the sight of the Lord. He is never to take wine or other fermented drink, and he will be filled with the Holy Spirit even before he is born. He will bring back many of the people of Israel to the Lord their God. And he will go on before the Lord, in the spirit and power of Elijah, to turn the hearts of the parents to their children and the disobedient to the wisdom of the righteous – to make ready a people prepared for the Lord.

What a word of prophecy for a baby-to-be! Of course, the child they had waited for over the course of many years would be a "joy and a delight!"

Elizabeth's response when she became pregnant is documented in Luke 1:25. I have enjoyed reading her response in various Bible translations.

> "The Lord has done this for me," she said. "In these days He has shown His favor and taken away my disgrace among the people." (NIV)

> "So, this is how God acts to remedy my unfortunate condition!" she said. (The Message)

> "How kind the Lord is," she exclaimed, "to take away my disgrace of having no children!" (The Living Bible)

Culturally, it was a disgrace for women to not be able to bear children (especially sons). But I believe that along with the societal pressure they faced, each of these women that I mention had a desire in their hearts to be a mama. There are still many women living in the United States and in other countries who come from a cultural background where they face a similar stigma when they do not have children. The Lord saw and knew the cultural disgrace that Elizabeth faced by not having children. He also saw the longing in her heart. He was so kind to answer her prayers with a baby.

One more reason I love this story about Elizabeth is because my given name is Elizabeth. The words about Elizabeth that Gabriel said to Mary spoke to me very personally several months ago, as found in Luke 1:36-37 (1984 NIV): "Even Elizabeth your relative is going to have a child in her old age, and she who was said to be barren is in her sixth month. For nothing is impossible with God."

I'm not old, but technically according to the medical definition, at this point I'm barren. I have a womb that has not yet produced life, no matter what I have tried. Elizabeth had never conceived and she was post-menopausal. The angel told Mary that she would be the mother of Jesus, and mentioned that her cousin Elizabeth was pregnant in her old age. To me it seems that Gabriel casually ended his statement with: "For nothing is impossible with God."

My dream of having babies of my own is not impossible with God.

One more insight I want to share about Elizabeth was beautifully written by my friend Amy Frank. She wrote this on Facebook in December 2013 after reading an Advent devotional:

> I don't think I ever put it together before that the angel's appearance to Zechariah in the temple was the break in the 400 years of silence between the testaments. Tell me God doesn't care about our everyday personal lives; He chose to break His silence by addressing a barren couple's prayer for a child.

People had not directly heard God's voice for generations – at least not which had been recorded in the Bible. The Old Testament prophets had come and gone, with a yet unfulfilled promise of Jesus who would later come with healing, salvation, and restoration.

Before Mary received her message from Gabriel, Zechariah, a faithful priest, had gone into the temple to perform his ceremonial duties. There for the first time in hundreds of years, a person heard God's voice – and God told this old man that his old wife was going to have a baby!

After hearing from God that a baby was coming, Elizabeth conceived and had a baby despite her age! Their son John was the passionate preacher who prepared the way for Jesus' ministry. Jesus even said of John in Matthew 11:11: "Truly I tell you, among those born of women there has not risen anyone greater than John the Baptist..."

John was vital in God's plan for Jesus' time here on earth, and therefore John's birth was intended for a specific time. Although Elizabeth might have hoped to have a baby decades earlier, it is clear that God's timing was right.

This story gives me hope that there might likewise be a reason (still unrecognized by me) as to why my children haven't come sooner.

Samson's Mother

In addition, there is Samson's mother, whose name we do not know. Judges 13:2–3 says:

> A certain man... had a wife who was childless, unable to give birth. The angel of the Lord appeared to her and said, "You are barren and childless, but you are going to become pregnant and give birth to a son."

She and her husband had some conversations and interactions with the angel of God, including asking God how they should raise this promised son. Just as the angel said, she gave birth to Samson, who was blessed by God and used by Him to destroy the enemy.

Once again, God brought forth from a barren woman a special child to accomplish His purposes.

Hannah

The name Hannah is popular these days, and I find it interesting that so many Hannahs and Samuels I meet are the first child conceived or adopted after a period of barrenness. Hannah in the Bible is remembered for demonstratively crying out to God for a child.

Though it's hard for me to imagine these dynamics, Hannah and another woman were both married to the same husband, and 1 Samuel 1:2–5 says that Peninnah (the other wife) had children, but Hannah had none, because the Lord had closed her womb.

That alone is complicated. As I'm working my way through the Old Testament, there are times when God closes wombs as a curse or punishment. Yet there are women like Hannah whose wombs are closed for no apparent reason. I can relate. I don't know of any specific reason why God has not yet allowed my womb to be fruitful, nor is there any clear medical or spiritual reason that we have found. I can imagine how much more difficult my journey would be if my husband had another wife who had lots of babies. That's one of the many reasons I'm glad that we don't live in a polygamist society!

Poor Hannah, she was loved by her husband, but I'm not sure he was the most sensitive man. 1 Samuel 1:8 says that "Elkanah her husband would say to her, 'Hannah, why are you weeping? Why don't you eat? Why are you downhearted?"

And he would ask, "Don't I mean more to you than ten sons?" My husband occasionally says that to me in jest. Unlike my husband, I presume that Hannah's spouse was serious. Thankfully, Mike is sensitive enough to not make that joke when I am feeling down!

Now Hannah and her family would travel year after year to a place called Shiloh to worship. 1 Samuel 1:10 says that on one of those trips, "In her deep anguish Hannah prayed to the Lord, weeping bitterly." I have wondered if she was extra emotional due to being close to her period. Maybe she was crying so much because of grief and hormones, or maybe her grief alone was enough to cause her to be distraught.

When Eli the priest saw her, he thought she was drunk. When he realized she was just praying, he said, "Go in peace, and may the God of Israel grant you what you have asked of Him." (1 Samuel 1:17)

What words of hope, peace, and encouragement to hear from a minister, a prophet, a man who speaks the word of God! The Bible says that Hannah and her husband came together intimately, and that God remembered her. Had God forgotten her when He closed her womb? I doubt that our loving and all-knowing Father actually forgot her, but in that holy moment, God allowed a baby to be formed. Finally, Hannah conceived and then gave birth to her son whom she named Samuel, which means, "Asked of God."

Hannah had promised God that if He would give her a baby, then she would give him back to the Lord. So once Samuel was weaned, he went to live in the temple with Eli, and Samuel, like many other long-awaited babies, went on to do mighty things in the kingdom of God.

The Shunammite Woman

The Shunammite woman, as we know her, was a woman who provided warm hospitality to Elisha, a prophet in the Old Testament. One day, as recorded in 2 Kings 4:14–17, Elisha wanted to return kindness for her hospitality, so he asked,

> "What can be done for her?" Gehazi [his servant] said, "She has no son, and her husband is old." Then Elisha said, "Call her." So he called her, and she stood in the doorway.

> "About this time next year," Elisha said, "you will hold a son in your arms." "No, my lord!" she objected. "Please, man of God, don't mislead your servant!" But the woman became pregnant, and the next year about that same time she gave birth to a son, just as Elisha had foretold.

It certainly can be hard to receive words of hope when we're in a hopeless place. Sarah laughed at the idea of becoming pregnant at her age. The Shunammite woman's response was more of a plea: "No, don't get my hopes up!" I know that feeling.

I look at this woman and I relate to her desire, her feelings of not wanting false hope, and I see that God is faithful, even if we don't always respond to Him in faith.

The Bleeding Woman

Although the Bible doesn't say that this woman was specifically dealing with infertility, and it does not mention her family, I feel like her story applies to many of us struggling to have a baby. Luke 8:43–48 describes a woman who had been bleeding for twelve years. She had sought medical help but nobody could heal her. One day, as Jesus was walking through a crowd, she reached out and touched the edge of His robe, and immediately she was healed. Jesus said, "Daughter, your faith has healed you. Go in peace."

After trying to conceive for several years, and after nearly twenty years of painful periods, I was diagnosed with endometriosis. I joined an endometriosis support group online and realized that compared to many others, my symptoms are mild. Many women who struggle with not being able to conceive a child also have some wacky stuff going on with their menstrual cycles, when I read this verse I realized two things: Jesus cares about us individually in our pain, bleeding, and desperation, and He responds to our faith.

Mike and I pray regularly for our bodies to be healed of whatever is keeping us from conceiving. We are not 100 percent sure what the issue is that holds us back, but we have sought medical care, and we ask God to heal.

In those months when I'm bleeding for ten days, wondering what the remedy is to make my menstrual cycle work like the textbooks say it ought to, I can reach out to God. He created me and He cares about me. When my cycle leaves me feeling not-so-sexy or fertile, I remember that God cares enough to include in the Bible this story of a woman with a bleeding disorder who is healed by Jesus.

Simeon

I also want to mention a man who waited for a miracle baby. Luke 2:25–35 tells the story of Simeon, who was a godly man awaiting the consolation of Israel. The Holy Spirit was upon him and had showed him that he would not die before he saw the Messiah. On the day that Joseph and Mary brought baby Jesus into the temple, Simeon picked Him up and praised God.

Simeon had waited for many years to set his eyes on a certain miracle baby. I wonder if people knew that he was waiting. I wonder if those around him thought he was crazy for thinking he would see this promise come to pass in his lifetime. Did he look like a fool, day after day watching and waiting for this promise to become reality?

Sometimes I wonder if people think that the stance of hope, faith, and expectation that Mike and I are taking is foolish. Don't people say that insanity is doing the same thing over and over and expecting a different outcome? Do people think we're crazy for waiting and still hoping?

Simeon heard from God. He had faith in God's promise. He watched and waited.

The One for whom Simeon waited would be the consolation of Israel. Obviously, our future child will not be Jesus. Our child, however, will be a gift from God. And in a sense, our child will be a consolation, which Webster defines as a "comfort received by a person after a loss or disappointment." Our future child will bring comfort to our empty arms – in the end we will not be disappointed.

Women in the Lineage of Jesus

There are five women mentioned in the bloodline of Christ. Upon reading the stories of these women, I noticed a common thread among the first four: Tamar, Rahab, Ruth, and Bathsheba. All of these women were married or in sexual relationships, yet the Bible does not provide evidence that they conceived children in those relationships. Then later, when God's timing was right, each of those women was married or in a relationship (Tamar's story is rather complex) with God's intended man, and through that marriage or relationship she bore a son. These were all ancestors of Joseph, the earthly father of Jesus. Although the Bible doesn't explicitly state that these women were unable to bear children earlier in their lives, it's implied that for some reason they were not fertile until God's timing was right because He intended a certain child to be born at a certain time.

God gives miracle babies both to the pure and to the prostitute. Rebekah was a virgin when she got married, and her miracle twins were born twenty years into her marriage. Rahab was a prostitute, and the Bible doesn't mention if she had any pregnancies during those years. However, God rescued her and then allowed her to marry an Israelite, one of His chosen people, which was a highly unusual exception. God then gave her a son who became part of the lineage of Jesus. I believe that regardless of a person's sexual past, if that person's heart is repentant toward God, their sin is forgiven. God is able to make all things new and He is the giver of miracle babies.

The reality is that all of the couples mentioned in these past two chapters struggled with childlessness and lack of pregnancy as my husband and I do. They didn't have modern medicine or ovulation predictor kits. They likely had some degree of knowledge about medicine and herbs. (For example, Genesis 30:14 says that Rachel wanted to buy Leah's mandrakes, a plant used to boost fertility.) Like us, these women had desire, and they had lack; but they also had God and they had faith in Him. He did miracles, gave them babies, and He intended for those babies to become mighty men in God's kingdom.

As I study these women in the Bible who battled barrenness, I am encouraged. These women eventually had supernatural pregnancies. Sarah, Rebekah, Rachel, Hannah, and Elizabeth probably thought at times that they might never have babies of their own. Their only option was asking God and waiting, and He heard and answered.

When a person has nothing but God to rely on, then that person fully depends on Him.

I live in a world where it seems that I can do anything I want. I can pursue almost any career, I can live anywhere I want, and I can acquire information about anything on the internet. Yet I strive to do something that seemingly should be uncomplicated: become pregnant.

After two surgeries, a year of fertility medicine, utilizing technology to understand my fertility, and doing everything in my power to conceive, I am still not pregnant.

When all is said and done, the only One I can turn to is God. These women didn't have the options that we have; all they had was a husband, time, and God.

Eventually God created new life in their barren wombs. It all comes down to His timing and purpose.

The sons that these women gave birth to became men who were key to the history of our Christian faith, and many were the direct ancestors of Jesus! Isaac, Jacob, Judah, Joseph, Samuel, John – what if their mamas had given up? What if they had quit praying? What if they had let their marriages die due to the pain of childlessness? What if they had settled for alternative options and then stopped there, instead of being open to God's plan?

What about those who have faith that God will give them babies, but He doesn't? Hebrews 11:13 mentions, "All these people were still living by faith when they died. They did not receive the things promised; they only saw them and welcomed them from a distance." There are people who live by faith until they die, not receiving what they are believing for, but they hold on until the end. My hope and desire is that I will believe God's promises for my life even to the grave.

This battle for fertility has been fought before; it's not a new problem. I am encouraged by this great cloud of witnesses who went before us, who saw God's miracle power in pregnancy then bore children, because nothing is impossible with God.

Chapter 10 – My Crowd of Witnesses

I was running
then two people cheered for me
and I ran faster.

Sydney, age 5
when describing a race at kindergarten

As I have vulnerably shared with people that we have been trying to conceive, I find myself surrounded, not just by a spiritual *cloud* of witnesses as referred to in Hebrews 12, but also by my own *crowd* of witnesses here on earth.

This crowd is made up of people who are eagerly watching, encouraging, praying, and sending me emails filled with words of hope. Even if there are some in the crowd who are gossiping, judging, and critiquing, I have a feeling that this crowd of witnesses will cheer me on in this race of endurance and will surround me when I get to the finish line. God has designed us to live in community, and He intends that when any of us share our struggles in a healthy way, we won't be ridiculed; we'll be supported.

Fertility challenges encompass private matters such as health, reproductive organs, sex life, and finances. Come to think of it, this subject even touches on those personal topics of politics and religion, right? Not many people discuss these topics freely, yet they are intimately tied to a couple's inability to conceive.

Since our friends and family know that we're trying to have a baby, occasionally people will ask if there is any news. Because we share openly about our situation, it is okay for people to ask, although it can be awkward. No news basically means no baby yet.

Because I have talked rather freely about the fact that I have been trying to become pregnant for such a long time, I have found myself surrounded by others struggling to grow their family. Some friends have faced secondary infertility; after having a child or two, they intended to expand their families only to discover that it's not happening easily. I used to feel alone with this issue, but now I find that I meet people all the time who are struggling to have a baby.

I have since realized that the enemy of our souls wants to create and promote this feeling of isolation in us. He knows that if we don't share with others, we cannot help them, and they cannot help us. The truth is, we're not alone.

Social media makes the fertility struggle bittersweet. It can easily be a place where I am constantly reminded of what I lack. My Facebook newsfeed is filled with pictures of babies and birth announcements. On one particular day, a friend announced their fourth baby in four years while another added one hundred pictures of her newborn baby's second day out of the womb. (One hundred photos. From the child's second day in the hospital.) Girls who I used to babysit now have children of their own. And here I am, well into my thirties, married, stable, ready for children, but with empty arms.

On the flip side social media can connect people. I remember browsing through an array of "what I'm thankful for in November" Facebook posts to see a childhood friend's statement that she was so glad her parents kept trying to have children even when doctors said they wouldn't be able to. Because Jamie's parents didn't give up, she and her brother were born. Other friends have shared testimonies of the faithfulness of God to bring them children, even after years of trying. Glimpses of these encouraging stories, even on Facebook, fill my empty heart with hope. I privately thanked Jamie for sharing those words, then many months later she sent me a message out of the blue: "You have crossed my mind lately. I am still praying for you and that God gives you the desires of your heart! Just wanted to tell you." This is someone I haven't seen face-to-face since we played basketball together in eighth grade – yet through modern ways of communication God has used her to encourage me.

More than once I have checked my Facebook and found words of encouragement through private Facebook messages. Many of these are from people that I don't know very well in real life, but as we have connected online they have seen my blog writings about our fertility journey, and God has reminded these women to pray for me and encourage me. More than once, these words have come at just the right time and my bitter tears have turned sweeter. I know that God knows my heart, and He wants me to be encouraged.

Kristen, a friend-of-a-friend whom I have only met briefly, sent me a message one night as I was lying in bed feeling sorry for myself because I had just started my period:

> "Hi Betsy, hope you are well. I wanted to let you know that God had laid you on my heart to pray for. I don't know you very well at all, but something about your struggle with infertility really touched my heart. In the past few days I have felt led to pray more for you and to share a verse that helped me when Stan and I were waiting for one of our babies. *Habakkuk 2:3 For the revelation awaits an appointed time; it speaks of the end and will not prove false. Though it linger, wait for it; it will certainly come and will not delay.* God's ways are hard to understand, but always good. I am praying for patience and peace while you wait for God to reveal His plan for your family. Blessings to you."

It was so timely and encouraging to me that God decided to speak to a near-stranger in another town and prompt her to both pray for me as well as to send me an encouraging message. I'm thankful that she prayed and that she shared that Scripture with me, reminding me that God's timing is right.

My husband's cousin Pasaka has sent me many encouraging notes. She understands, because she also had to wait a while for her babies to come along and she now has three beautiful children. She remembered me this past Mother's Day, a day when I spent the afternoon and evening with puffy eyes red from tears. "For the littles you mother daily [as a nanny], for the babes that you'll (soon! Lord) hold in your arms and that will call you Mama – happy Mother's Day, sweet Betsy."

Another friend sent me a message beginning with, "When you have your baby..." I appreciate her choice of words – she knows of my dreams, and she said "when" because she believes that it will happen.

One morning I was awakened by a text message from an unfamiliar number: "Had a dream of you being seven months pregnant!" I looked at it, went back to sleep, and then later during the day wondered who it was from. When I sent a text back later in the day to ask who my mysterious messenger was, it turned out to be my dear friend who was texting from a different phone number. God knew that it was just the time of the month when I needed that word of encouragement, so I choose to believe that my friend's dream is a glimmer of hope, a prophetic dream that God does indeed have a baby for us.

Not only has social media provided a network of people experiencing similar struggles, but talking to people in real life and mentioning that we've tried for a long time to conceive has knitted my heart together with other people and bolstered my confidence that God is in the midst of this.

I'm grateful for the people I cross paths with just long enough for words of encouragement or prayers of faith. One time I went to get a haircut while I was traveling, and the stylist and I chatted while she cut my hair. Before I left her shop that day she reached her hand out to my midsection and prayed for my womb.

A friend who is a grandmother now but remembers her own wait for babies told me recently that while traveling in Rome, she lit a candle for me and prayed for me in a cathedral there. I loved hearing that she was thinking of me and praying specifically for my babies-yet-to-come during her travels.

Sometimes I stand in my closet, searching for a different outfit to wear, and I see maternity clothes tucked in the back, waiting patiently for me. I feel thankful for the friends who finished having babies and passed their maternity clothes on to me in faith that I will one day need them. More than one family has handed over their baby items to us, and some are even saving the baby items they no longer need, with expectation that we will one day use them for babies of our own. Their actions demonstrate faith that one day our children will come.

Mike and I are grateful for our supportive parents and family members, for friends and acquaintances, for those who have walked this road before us. We have been encouraged by many people. A pastor shared with Mike that it had taken him and his wife several years to become pregnant with their first child, and now twenty-some years later they can clearly see that God's timing was right.

These crowds of witnesses, cheering us on in unison or one by one, help us get through our challenges. Lynette Lewis, an author and speaker, shared an illustration one day when I heard her speak. She told of a time when she had watched the New York City Marathon as the runners came through Central Park. Toward the end of the race she saw some people with their names painted on the front of their shirts. Her first thought, being a fashion-conscious woman, was something along the lines of, "How cheesy! Why would someone wear their name on their shirt?" Then she heard the bystanders cheering for these runners individually, "Go, George!" "C'mon Joanne, you can do it!" She realized that those runners knew that by wearing their names across their chests they would receive encouragement.

While writing this book, I ran my first half marathon. The race that I participated in was a "Run Like a Diva" half marathon. It took place on an overcast, cool September morning, which was ideal weather for a race. Despite the cloudy skies I ran those thirteen miles with my sunglasses perched on top of my head just in case the sun came out. Nearing the finish line I thought about how I hadn't needed sunglasses for a moment, yet keeping them close on a cloudy day demonstrates faith. I believed that the sun would come out again, therefore I kept my shades with me. Faith is believing that the sun will come out again, even when clouds cover the sky. Faith is believing that God is able to give us children, even when it doesn't seem possible.

For obvious reasons, the vast majority of people running the "Run Like a Diva" half marathon were women. Looking around at the crowd as we ran, I saw many women who looked like runners – they had fit bodies and they seemed to know what they were doing. Yet there were even more women who did not look like runners, but they had determination on their faces and their feet carried them through a 13.1 mile course – sometimes faster and sometimes slower.

As we took off from the starting line there was a surge of adrenaline – and quite the surge of estrogen as this crowd of people clad in pink tutus, tiaras, and sparkles began to run. There was energy and excitement in the air. A few miles into the race we began to experience our first hills and adversity began to hit us as our bodies became tired and our minds became aware of the ascent and the distance.

Around that point in the race, I began to feel choked up with emotion. Tears were threatening to sneak out of my eyes – and I didn't want to be seen crying while I ran!

I felt emotional because I so deeply understood that life is like a big race – and having people around us to cheer us on is vital! We often feel like we're alone yet God has impressed upon my heart the concept that I am surrounded. I'm surrounded by that "great cloud of witnesses." Just like I'm not the only woman to run a half marathon, I'm not the only woman whose body won't get pregnant (yet). In these past few years God has placed woman after woman in my path who are going through the same issue, and my desire is to encourage them (as well as others that I will never meet) with some of the hope that God has given to me.

So as I ran the course, I felt emotional knowing that I was not struggling through this race alone – nearly two thousand other women were putting one foot in front of the other on their way to the finish line. I was surrounded by people in that same demanding position that I was in.

During this race, I was grateful for the clusters of people along the way cheering us on. As we ran from the country road into the residential neighborhoods, people came out onto their front porches and dragged chairs to their driveways to sit and watch us. Many people held up handmade signs to encourage us and I went out of my way to give the little kids a high five. Overall, I felt supported in this race by total strangers even if some of them were leisurely eating their breakfasts as we ran by.

In our journey to start a family, Mike and I have shared with people that we are hoping for a baby. When we open up about this sensitive topic, people can see that we're running hard after our goal. People cheer us along, pray for us, and support us with words of hope and encouragement. That helps so much! Knowing that there are people believing, praying, and cheering us on keeps me going. If you do not find yourself surrounded by encouraging people, perhaps you can begin opening up to people who are safe to share your struggle with.

As we ran, we discovered that our course had tougher hills than what we expected. Another thought that floated through my head as I chugged along was that if it were up to me, I'd pick a different course. That is so much like my life. I would pick a different route with less challenging hills to climb, and my babies would have been born in my own planned time. This Scripture became more real to me as I ran:

Hebrews 12:1–2 (1984 NIV) says:

Therefore, since we are surrounded by such a great cloud of witnesses, let us throw off everything that hinders and the sin that so easily entangles, and let us run with perseverance the race marked out for us. Let us fix our eyes on Jesus, the author and perfecter of our faith, who for the joy set before Him endured the cross, scorning its shame, and sat down at the right hand of the throne of God.

In that half marathon, as I ran longer and harder than ever before, on a course that I did not choose, I was thankful to be one of many. Looking around, beyond my own circumstances and feelings, I realized that I was in the middle of a sea of women dealing with the same struggle, and on the sidelines was a crowd cheering me on!

That is so much like my journey to conceive a baby. I am surrounded. I'm going to run with perseverance. For the joy set before me, I will endure!

And yes, in a manner of speaking, I'll wear my name on my shirt, I'll be transparent and share my disappointing and challenging quest to have a baby if that means I'll be encouraged along the way.

One day Lynette Lewis spoke on the topic of "The Agony, the Ecstasy, and the Boring In Between." She has experienced these emotions, having waited many years for a husband, then adopting newborn twins later in life. Not long after her twin daughters joined her family, one of her stepsons passed away after a fight with cancer. In light of the grief and joy she has experienced she says, "Those who surround you in your agonies don't want to miss it when your ecstasy comes."

Lynette has faced delayed dreams and the grief of loss; yet I have witnessed her joy when those dreams are fulfilled in God's timing. In her book *Remember the Roses*, she writes that she feared that her wedding would be anticlimactic to those around her. However she discovered that everyone was more than excited to celebrate because they wanted to rejoice with her after her long wait. The same thing happened when her babies came many years later; she and her husband were extraordinarily showered with gifts as people celebrated the birth of God-given baby girls. Lynette truly knows that those who walk through the valleys with you will rejoice when you reach the mountaintop.

While initially it seemed scary and intimidating, I have found that sharing my struggle with safe and supportive people has allowed me to freely share it with strangers. This has gotten easier over time, even to the point where I am now writing about it publicly. By letting people see me "run this race," I realized that I have gained a support network that has strengthened me and I am in turn able to encourage others.

While running my half marathon, I was encouraged by the people who cheered for me. At the same time, while I ran I also chose to seize the opportunity to cheer others on. I spoke encouraging words to a woman in her sixties as I ran alongside her for a few minutes. It benefits all parties when we encourage others. Reaching out to other women and trying to draw them out of isolation and into community strengthens all of us. The enemy of our souls wants to wreck our lives and steal our joy, and one of the ways that he tries to achieve this goal is by making us feel isolated and vulnerable. We are stronger in community, our hearts, emotions, and spirits are protected there.

Friends. Family. Mere acquaintances and people I haven't seen in 20 years sending me Facebook messages to let me know that they're praying. The hairdresser. People I know well and those that I only met once are cheering me on, letting me know that I am not alone in this journey. Not only is God for me (not against me), but He has provided people to support me along the way.

Truly, I am surrounded.

As little Sydney said at the beginning of the chapter, *when people cheer, we run faster*.

Chapter 11 – When God Speaks

Blessed is she who believed that there would be
a fulfillment of what was spoken to her from the Lord.
Luke 1:45 (ESV)

God has not only encouraged us through Scripture's cloud of witnesses and through the people cheering us on, but He has also surprised us with images in nature and words of reassurance.

We live in the suburbs of Washington, DC, home of the Cherry Blossom Festival. In the springtime, the trees around here bloom with flowers unlike anything I have ever seen. Flowering trees in all hues of pink, purple, and white fill the neighborhoods. Several times this past spring as I was driving around gazing at the trees, I noticed that among the beautiful blooming foliage there stood big desolate-looking trees. Those trees stood out against the sky like fleshless skeletons – no leaves, flowers, or evidence of life could be seen. I sensed the Holy Spirit whispering this phrase to my heart: *just because it looks barren doesn't mean that it is.*

I knew that this applied to my fertility. Just because I'm not blooming with a pregnant belly, just because I don't have that maternal glow, and just because I've had no pregnancies yet does not mean that my womb is dead. Just because it looks dead doesn't mean that there is no life yet to come forth.

In the weeks following, I watched those late-blooming trees as tiny green leaves appeared. I kept my eye on them as they demonstrated that they were not lifeless, they were not barren, empty, skeletons. There was life inside – it just appeared later than the surrounding trees. Just because it looks barren doesn't mean that it will never bring forth life. Somehow, despite my circumstances, it is possible to believe that new life can come from my body.

As I wait for my babies to even be conceived I have meditated on Jeremiah 1:5 where God says: "Before I formed you in the womb, I knew you."

At this point in my writing, we've been trying for more than four years to get pregnant. Four years is equivalent to an entire presidential term, all the years that an average kid is in high school, and it's long enough for some of my friends to have had two or three babies. It's enough time for a woman to be disappointed more than 50 times, reminded by her body again and again that she is not pregnant.

Needless to say, I think about my future babies and pray incessantly for God to bring them into our lives. For me, they're just a hope, yet *God already knows my children*. Already. He knows their genders, their names, their destinies and callings, and He knows exactly why they will be born at specific times. He understands the delay of their conception. I will continue to pray for them, and I am so reassured to know that their Creator already knows them. Truthfully, I can't fully comprehend that.

And I am grateful for a God who speaks.

I remember a certain cold February night in 2012, climbing out of my husband's favorite old BMW in the parking lot of the campus of our rival university. We had arrived at North Carolina State University to watch their wrestling team compete against the University of North Carolina. Although I never attended UNC, my husband and my parents did, so it's the team we root for.

Since it was so close to Valentine's Day, going to a wrestling match with my husband practically counted as a date. This was only the second wrestling match I had ever watched, but I found that once a spectator can mentally get past the nearly indecent wrestling attire, watching a match is quite interesting. To me it looks painful, yet it's a show of great strength. Those same words describe this season of not being able to get pregnant: we're wrestling with it. It's painful. And it's a show of strength, although the strength doesn't come from us. Instead, as we wait upon the Lord, He renews our strength.

The wrestling match ended, and since we were in Raleigh already, we decided to stop by a local church that was hosting international guest speakers whose ministry we appreciated. Back in 2008 we had gone to this same church on our second date to hear this husband and wife team preach and prophesy, so that particular church holds good memories. Especially hopeful and encouraging to us that night was the fact that this was a very highly respected, internationally known pastoral couple.

Prophecy is the biblical practice of God speaking through one person to another in order to strengthen, encourage, and comfort them (see 1 Corinthians 14:3). Prophets are people who are gifted by God with these prophetic words, and this husband and wife team are very respected in the Christian community. The New Testament says to test a prophecy to make sure that it is accurate. In my experience, more times than not the prophetic words I have received have been true.

In fact, I distinctly remember a prophetic word I received four years before meeting Mike, where the prophet told me, "The Lord's in no hurry." Knowing my impatience in life, my friends and I laughed when we heard that. Without a doubt, the Lord was speaking to me about my future that night!

After the wrestling match, we drove across town and slipped into the back of the church just as the sermon was wrapping up. Shortly thereafter, the minister began walking around the sanctuary sharing prophetic words with the people that God directed him toward. When he walked in our direction, I hoped that God would direct him to share something with us, as I always desire encouragement from the Lord. Sure enough, he walked right up to us and asked us to stand up.

He began to share some good things from the heart of God for us. Then he said to me (italics are added for emphasis and what is in brackets are my comments):

> "You know dear, I love the Spirit of the Lord that is all over you and the Lord says you know, this isn't going to

be the season of disappointment [tears filled my disappointed eyes] but this is going to be the season of breakthrough..."

He interrupted himself to ask us: "You guys got kids? Where are they?"

I replied with a shake of the head and a "not yet."

"Oh you don't have kids yet, oh sorry. You know there are kids coming very soon."

I interjected by saying, "Good!" Then I laughed nervously and others in the church chuckled.

"Yeah, there are kids coming soon and you know guys, I see, as I came up and I saw you I kept seeing children over and over and over, you know – and *it wasn't just other people's children* it was your own children. And I see there's breakthrough coming up in that area and the Lord says He's heard your cries and He has heard the word that you guys have spoken out. And I want you to know that this is not the season of disappointment, but this is going to be a season of seeing the reward of the Lord. Remember when I told you about fruitfulness when I walked up here, yeah, that's one of the fruits that God is coming to bring over the two of you. And you're going to see that breakthrough. And you know, the word of men is not the word of God, amen?"

Oh. My. Goodness. His words resonated in my heart. Of course they would be meaningful! My heart soared when this man of God said that he looked at us and saw "children – not just other people's children but our own children." I knew that God was encouraging me personally. Could he have known that at that point in my life, I was an aunt, a regular babysitter, and one who just adored the children in my life? He did not know that I spent a lot of time loving children who were not my own. I believe that God wanted me to know that I would have my own children.

God knew back in February 2012 how desperately I wanted children. God spoke hope into my circumstances. And as I type this, it's 2014, and a printout of that prophetic word stares back at me from the front of our refrigerator. For more than two years when I've walked through my kitchen, when I have stood before those words with tears in my eyes and menstrual cramps gripping my body, I have reminded myself of God's promise to me.

And that was not the first prophetic word I received on that matter, nor was it the last. In the summer of 2011 (more than a year after we began trying to conceive) another internationally known prophet visited our church in Durham. I remember nervously walking into a Saturday afternoon teaching and prayer session, where Pastor Willem of South Africa was teaching about healing and praying for people.

After he finished teaching, he started out the prayer time by having those of us in the room pray for one another. One young woman from the church who I didn't know very well looked at me and began, "Well, I'm not sure if this is okay to say…" I encouraged her to go for it, whatever it was. "When I look at you right now I just hear one word: Children." Tears came. "That's why I'm here today," I replied, and a short time later when I asked Pastor Willem to pray for me he said that he had prayed for women all over the world to have babies, and they had babies. Then he prayed for me. He's my Facebook friend to this day so that I can contact him with good news when my time comes.

God continually speaks words of hope to us as we ask Him for a child.

One would think that in four years, I probably would have had a conversation with God about why we are not yet pregnant. I've talked over the whys with Mike time and time again. I almost wonder that if I approach God with that question, that He will tell me an answer that I really don't like. What if He says it's because of something that I have done or not done? Scarier still would be if He answered with "because you or Mike are going to die soon." Or "you're not going to have children." Will God give me an answer that I just can't handle?

Even as I write this, I see how fear has had a grip on my heart as I approach this subject.

I began to ask God the "why" question, and the first answer that I felt He impressed on my heart is simply because it's not His time yet. That's what my husband has been saying all along – as we've asked of God, we sense that our promised children will come – in His timing.

Another woman in my great crowd of witnesses is a friend I met in the waiting room of the OB/GYN office. It's an unusual place to begin a friendship, but Mike spotted her across the room because he recognized her from our church worship team. I started a conversation with Jacki, and a friendship was formed. I was in the office that day for a pre-op appointment, as I was having surgery for endometriosis the following week. She later told me that she was there that day to confirm her pregnancy with her first baby.

Nearly a year later we were together at a social event, and she stepped away for a time to nurse her baby. When she came back she shared a vision that the Lord had given her for Mike and me. She saw us together, united, on the hand of a clock, and the clock hand was approaching the right time. She said that it was like God was saying that we were close, almost to that right time.

Prophetic words must be weighed according to the Scripture. If these words do not line up with what God says in His written word, they are not from Him. Yet the Bible makes it clear that reproduction is His design and that He sees couples having children as a good thing.

In this season we're doing our part to try to conceive a baby. We're trusting that God will bless us with a child when His time is right, and we desire to walk through this season with grace.

One day, as Mike and I were driving several hours back to our home after visiting family in North Carolina, I shared some thoughts with him. I told him about a comment that I heard Pastor Bill Johnson say in a sermon podcast.

The phrase that stuck out to me from that particular sermon was that he had prayed "that his children would not live in frustration as he had."

Why did that resonate so loudly inside of me? Because I have lived so much of my life in frustration. In my wait for a husband I clung to the idolization of marriage and forfeited God's grace for that season. I was frustrated as a single woman. I felt discontent in most of my jobs in the first decade out of college. I was certainly irritated when plans didn't go as I preferred. I have seen frustration in some of my family members, and I've been frustrated a lot in my own life. I don't want our children to live in needless frustration.

When I heard his prayer for the next generation to not live in frustration, it hit home. I agreed in prayer that our offspring would not live in frustration. Interestingly enough, since then, my level of frustration with the things of this life has dissipated. I'm just not as frustrated as I used to be, and I refuse to pass that trait on to the next generation. One way to overcome frustration is to live in an attitude of thankfulness – which Mike and I try to do now and is something we intend to teach to our children. The devil is the only one who should live in frustration, because he's never going to win.

During that same car trip with Mike, I commented about how three close friends had just asked me if I was wallowing in sadness and grief regarding not being able to have babies yet. To summarize all three friends, they basically said, "I'm so sad for you... you can grieve you know... and are you sure you're not wallowing when nobody's looking?"

It's true that in the first six months of dealing with our fertility struggle, I was pretty sad. Around the two year mark my hope was pretty dim and my faith was running low. Yet in recent months I have not grieved nearly as much, I have not been very sad, and I haven't wallowed in despair, although not a day passes that I don't think about how much I want children. I told my husband a good reason why I'm not as distraught now as people might expect me to be: because I have been to the pit of despair. I visited there too often in my twenties. Feelings of depression, despair, and discouragement hung around me way too often. It was not a good place to be, so frankly, having been there, I am quite certain that I don't want to go back.

I am choosing instead to hang onto faith, hope, and a God who loves me, knowing that He will get me through.

Not only have we received encouraging words from gifted prophets, we have also received numerous words of hope from people all around us. A young woman who prayed for us at a church service one day, who did not know our circumstances, said she saw a picture from God of us with our children. A stranger who sat beside us one Sunday heard a piece of our story and prayed over us to have children. Over and over again God has provided people to stand with us in prayer and in faith that we would indeed have children.

Recently my mother-in-law, Lydia Herman, wrote me a letter after attending a ladies' retreat with her church. A speaker at the retreat had shared her story of having health problems and trying to conceive for years. Here is what she wrote to me:

> With one disappointment after another, Jennifer cried out to the Lord: "It has been so long! Why are my prayers still not answered?" And she felt the Holy Spirit saying: "Jennifer, the gift you seek is a child with his own destiny, so this is not just about your long wait. Your child has a purpose for his generation, and a specific time and place for his birth." Jennifer received that, and on their second attempt at in-vitro, their son was born. A few years later their twins were born as well.
>
> Jennifer's spiritual message to us that day was that it takes brave faith to keep trusting after a disappointment, and especially after a series of them. She said that when we see our plan A failing, remember this – God's plan B is always Better. Our view is narrow, like tunnel vision, but He sees what will be best for all concerned. So I just wanted to encourage you, Betsy, as you wait for your prayers to be answered. This is just act two in a three act play – the story is far from over. And God is all-wise and all-loving.

I believe that the Lord has spoken to Mike and me – that we will be parents, that I will be a mother. We believe that He intends for me to give birth to children. It's daunting to write so boldly when nothing has happened – I have not yet become pregnant. The voice that whispers "What if you're wrong?" taunts me even as I write. However, I want to be that woman who believes that God will fulfill the word that the Lord has spoken to her!

I'm writing this book in obedience to God's calling, believing that God knows what He is doing, and with the goal to encourage others who find themselves in this same circumstance or situation.

Another story of how God demonstrated to me how He can bring new life out of something seemingly dead happened a couple of years ago.

Many people have pets, such as a dog that they take on walks, a cat who rules the house, or a fish that does whatever fish do, I will admit that I don't have any pets... I have houseplants.

In my childhood home was an enormous house plant called a split leaf philodendron, which had been given to my mother as a gift way before I was born. Around the time that I graduated from college, the plant split into several smaller plants. My mom gave me one of the smaller plants that quickly grew to its full size, earning the nickname "The Man-Eating Plant." Each leaf was a foot or two long, so it took up a significant amount of space in my living room. This plant came with me when I moved to North Carolina, and it dominated our living room after Mike and I married.

Then came the winter when Mike and I put a good-sized Christmas tree in our small living room. Along with our furniture and the Man-Eating Plant, there was just no space left for people, or Christmas gifts, or anything at all! Something had to go. After considering the risk, we dared to move the Man-Eating Plant outside to our porch for the winter with the hope that it would survive until spring. I wrapped newspaper and plastic around the base of the plant hoping that it would retain some warmth.

Well, after the next cold frosty night, the once huge green leaves turned brown and drooped to the ground. My plant was not surviving the winter outside. I really felt sad about my loss.

Summer came, and we moved what appeared to be the dead stalk of the plant from the shaded patio to a sunny area. I had a little bit of hope that it might revive in the summer sun and grow new leaves. It sat there for a while, and I ignored it, focusing instead on my tomato plants

Then one day I noticed a little bit of life peeking out of the dirt in the container that once held my Man-Eating Plant. Out of the seemingly dead stump in the dry soil popped something that resembled a stalk of celery! But it was not celery – it was a new Man-Eating Plant! I was so excited to see new life! The tiny plant grew bigger and bigger! I was overjoyed that LIFE had sprung out of what had appeared to be dead!

One day Mike and I decided it was time to extricate the little plant from the root system. Thanks to his care and wisdom, Mike went to the store and bought a special saw so that we could carefully cut this baby plant out of the big one. We took the plant out of the pot, and while Mike was carefully pulling away the dirt and roots, he found another baby plant within the root system.

Then we found another. And another. At the end of our digging we realized that we had four little baby plants growing deep in the root system of our large and seemingly dead plant.

This happened a year or two into our season of trying to get pregnant. I truly felt like God was showing me through His creation that even when a situation seems dead, or hopeless, He is capable of giving new and abundant life.

When we moved away from that apartment we gave a couple of the plants away, but we held onto two small pots full of our thriving little Man-Eating Plants (thankfully they are smaller than their mother plant was!) We keep them inside in the winter and outside in the summer; always a reminder of the One who gives new life.

In our slow and challenging season of wanting a baby but not yet seeing our hope fulfilled, we are grateful to know a God who speaks His words of hope. He cares enough about me to speak to me in many ways. So I choose to stand in hope with the words of the life-giving-miracle-working God echoing in my heart. I choose to believe that one day I will experience the tangible fulfillment of what God has spoken to me.

Luke 1:45 (ESV) says, "Blessed is she who believed that there would be a fulfillment of what was spoken to her from the Lord." There's no questioning the context of this Scripture: it's about miracle babies. Regardless of the promises that the Lord has spoken to us, we are truly blessed when we believe that He will fulfill them. This particular statement was made by Elizabeth, pregnant with her miracle baby John. She said those words upon the arrival of her cousin Mary, pregnant with Jesus, the most supernatural baby of all. She was speaking hope and encouragement to Mary who might have felt nervous and scared about her unusual circumstances. Blessed is she who believes that there will be a fulfillment of what was spoken to her from the Lord.

God speaks in so many ways: through the Bible, by the gentle voice of the Holy Spirit, as well as through the people that He places in our lives. I even see God working in the nature He created, such as in the barren-looking trees I observed in the spring.

Psalm 21:2 says, "You have granted him his heart's desire and have not withheld the request of his lips." That Scripture was imprinted on the program for our wedding as a reminder that God answered my prayer for a husband. He was faithful to answer that request, and He will be faithful to complete the good work that He has begun.

Chapter 12 – Faithful to the End

Now faith is confidence in what we hope for
and assurance about what we do not see.
Hebrews 11:1

When I began writing this book, I dreamed of writing the final chapter about my miracle pregnancy that had finally come. I wanted to share about my struggle and my hope, and then finally have a positive pregnancy test.

As the first draft of my manuscript reached completion, I felt more than ready to be pregnant. Then it happened: my period was late, significantly later than it had ever been. I tried not to feel too optimistic, yet taking pregnancy tests day after day resulted in a negative answer each time. It eventually became clear to us that the medication I was taking to prolong my cycle was actually working, and although all the circumstances seemed to be ideal for me to be pregnant, I was not.

The ending to my story hasn't yet happened like I'd planned.

As a nanny, I often have to remind the little ones that I am in charge. God speaks to me the same way, gently saying, "I'm in charge, Betsy, you're not."

I remember that He is the one writing my life story, and He is always good.

As I wait, pray, and trust God for a miracle baby, I have discovered that I can still be productive during my wait. Doing something while waiting makes the time go by faster. It's like trying to read in a slow-moving checkout line and suddenly realizing that I've moved to the front of the line.

During my wait for a baby, I began blogging, then I wrote this book and began working on some others. I worked in my day job, first in an office, then as a nanny. I was the primary breadwinner for a couple of years while Mike earned a Master's degree. I lost weight and began running. I grew as a person and pursued my passions.

If I had birthed the children I planned when I had wanted, I'm pretty sure that I would not have accomplished many, if any, of these things. I wouldn't be who I am today if my babies had come when I had intended. Ultimately, I grew in my faith and in my relationship with the Lord as I repeatedly turned to Him during this season.

My youngest sister met her husband, married him, and is now expecting her first child, all within the years that I have been trying to conceive. I don't know why pregnancy comes quickly to one and slowly to another, but I choose to rejoice for others despite my own situation. Maybe my joy for my sister's pregnancy would be greater if I too were pregnant, but I'll admit, I'm pretty excited about my new nephew.

I am grateful to have grown up in a family that loves God, and I can say that from the time I was old enough to understand, I have aimed to trust God and to love Him. In these past few years of repeatedly knocking on the door of Heaven with my heart's greatest desire, I have gotten to know the King so much better.

My outlook on life has changed because now I can truly say that I trust that God is good. I know that He is fighting for me. I sincerely believe that He has good gifts in store for me. Just because I don't get what I want when I want it doesn't change God's heart toward me.

Earlier I shared of my visit to a South American juvenile detention center and how God clearly showed me that He is good regardless of circumstances. Since that day I have had ample opportunity to question God's goodness. But He told me that He is good, and He made it so clear to me that I will never forget.

As I wait to experience my greatest dream of being a mother, I still trust that God is good. My husband can attest that I don't spend every moment raving about how good God is and how right His timing is. Even though I have moments of complaining and crying, disbelief and doubt, I find that joy still comes in the morning. God told me that He is good. His written Word says that He is good. I have come to understand that even when He doesn't give me what I want when I want it, He is still good, and His timing is right. I have also learned that He is God and I am not.

Overall, this experience of not becoming a mom when I thought I would has definitely deepened my faith.

Hebrews 11:13 talks about those who "were still living by faith when they died. They did not receive the things promised; they only saw them and welcomed them from a distance."

I remember the first time that I earnestly prayed for someone who was dying of cancer. Our church congregation and many others were asking God to heal this man. I visited him in the hospital in his final days, I cried when I heard of his passing, and I grieved with his family at his funeral. During that time I found encouragement in Hebrews 11:13, understanding that sometimes we will pray for healing and the person dies, but that should not change our faith. Faith is something we live out until death.

Nothing is impossible with God, yet there is still no guarantee that He will give us a baby. I think that He will, but as a result of what I have learned in this journey I can rest more easily now, knowing that He's in charge.

Choosing hope month after month is only possible when I have faith that God can do anything. Trusting that He is always good keeps hope in perspective.

Hebrews 11:39–40 states: "These were all commended for their faith, yet none of them received what had been promised, since God had planned something better…"

That's what faith is all about: believing God, and if it ends up that He doesn't do what we're believing Him to do, we trust that He has a better plan.

Living by faith unto death is the kind of faith that God wants us to have. It's a faith that says: my body doesn't seem to be working, I'm getting older, and circumstances aren't making it likely that I will conceive, but I still believe that God can give me the fruit of my womb. He's the one who breathes life into dry places. He's the one who does miracles. He's the one Elizabeth was talking about when she said (my paraphrase): "Well, look at me! Old and pregnant! Nothing is impossible with God!"

There may be people whose prayers are answered through adoption. Although we are not pursuing it right now, I'm still for adoption. Some couples feel strongly that birthing a child is what God is calling them to pursue, and it is okay to ask God to fill your empty womb.

Many women desire to be mothers, yet they want to be married first, and marriage doesn't seem to be happening for them. God knows the desires of your heart, so keep asking Him. Continue hoping. Have faith, for nothing is impossible with God.

Based on everything I know about God and His word, His answer to the woman asking for a child is "Yes!"

I believe that we should live in expectation that He will answer these prayers with a "Yes!"

I can trust that God is creating a happy ending for this season of infertility. One of the key concepts that I'm clinging to is that Romans 8:28 says that God works all things together for the good of His people. I know that God loves me and I truly believe that He's going to work it all out.

As I referred to Abraham's story in my cloud of witnesses, I quoted the description of his faith in Romans 4:18, beginning with, "Against all hope, Abraham in hope believed." In verses 20–21 of that same chapter we read more about Abraham:

> He did not waver through unbelief regarding the promise of God, but was strengthened in his faith and gave glory to God, being fully persuaded that God had power to do what He had promised.

What I find most impressive and inspiring in this passage is that despite repeatedly experiencing a lack of success throughout many years, as decades passed Abraham's faith actually grew stronger. This is what I would like to see for my life as well.

Ephesians 6 describes how we should fight spiritual battles by wearing the armor of God. The phrase that runs through my mind these days is found in verse 13, which instructs that when we face adversity we need to stand our ground, and then "…having done all, to stand firm." (ESV) There comes a point where all I can do is stand firm with faith and hope, eyes fixed on God.

In this journey, I've learned what it means to hope in God when what I'm hoping for seems unlikely. I've chosen to live a life of faith, trusting in the goodness and ability of God, even if I never see my desired end result. After trying to conceive, seeking medical help, and crying out to God like Hannah, all I can do is to stand, trusting that He is still good.

I want to be one who stands in faith until the end. I dream that it can be said of me, like Elizabeth said to Mary in Luke 1:45, "Blessed is she who has believed that the Lord would fulfill His promises to her!"

Part 3 – My Practical Suggestions

Chapter 13 – How Do We Talk About It?

*Didn't people know how hard this was
without the probing questions, painful reminders,
and the unwanted advice and opinions given?*

*Sally M. Jones
Longing Heart; Empty Arms*

One afternoon at a birthday party for a friend's child, I heard someone ask one of those dreaded personal questions. My mom and my sister were visiting me that weekend, so they attended this party with me. There we met a friend of the hostess, who was there that day with her husband and two young children. My sister, who is not afraid to jump right into any conversation, straightforwardly asked the woman if they were going to have more children. "That's the plan," the woman replied vaguely.

My mom, my sister, and I discussed it in the car on the way home. "You shouldn't ask people such personal questions!" I said. My mom replied, "But that's how we find out about these things!" We then went on to speculate about whether this woman might already be pregnant but just not wanting to share her news with us as strangers. It turned out that our guess was right – the mutual friend mentioned a few weeks later that this woman was indeed pregnant.

Are you going to have more kids? When are you going to have more kids? Don't you want to have kids? These types of questions certainly dig into personal matters, yet those questions pop into my mind often when I am meeting new friends in their childbearing years. If I'm close enough in relationship I don't shy away from the topic, but I do resist the urge to ask strangers about their plans for a family.

Although I love babies and I'm quite curious about other people's families, I also know firsthand the awkwardness and pain that can arise when those questions are asked.

One winter afternoon I attended a baby shower, and I was feeling emotionally fragile. I made small talk throughout the party, and as the baby shower was coming to an end, I sat down for some comforting baby snuggles. As I was holding a friend's newborn daughter, a woman came up to me and cheerily asked: "So, are you and Mike thinking about starting a family any time soon?"

Although I don't remember my exact words, my response was snippy, if not downright rude, saying something like, "We've been trying for years."

She didn't know how to respond to my comment or to my tone of voice, and our conversation ended as abruptly as it had begun. Looking back, I wish I had reacted with greater grace, but my reaction has taught me a few things.

Spiritually, I want to be filled with God's peace so that I respond to similar situations in a grace-filled manner.

Practically, I prefer to tell people about my struggle preemptively, so that I do not become defensive when they inquire. It's easier for me to make it known that our lack of children is not by choice. I want people to know that my desire is to have children. I want to make it clear that we are doing what we can, and we are also waiting on the Lord.

Putting myself into this position proactively minimizes the negative emotions I feel when someone asks me when we're going to have kids. Instead of letting that question prick my heart every time, I prefer to make it known that we want children and that we welcome people to stand with us in prayer.

One of the most challenging factors in this already painful journey of trying to conceive is figuring out how to graciously respond to the (sometimes insensitive) comments from people who don't know what it's like.

Although I'm a nanny for a family that has four children and my days are full of little ones, I go home at night with a longing for my own babies. One day, when the youngest child was a few months old, we were at an event. I introduced myself to a woman there, explaining that I was the nanny for these children, and that my husband and I did not yet have children.

"Oh, I bet being a nanny is great birth control!" the woman replied.

Statements like that can be offensive, if not hurtful, to a woman who is doing everything she can to get pregnant. I informed the woman that we had actually been trying to have a baby, and the conversation quickly moved on.

In the early years of trying to start a family, I responded in many ways when asked about our plans for children. Initially I would tell people, "We're hoping to have a baby soon!" Eventually that became, "We hope God gives us a baby soon," or "We're waiting for God to give us a baby."

I've snapped at a few people, I've tried to playfully turn the conversation away from when I'll have a baby, and I've even commented that "No, I'm not pregnant, just fat." Maybe I should just say, "No, it's just a food baby."

One key that I try to keep in mind when innocent (but thoughtless) questions come is God's instruction for us to operate in grace and mercy towards others. I will admit that mercy is not one of my strong points, yet it's an area in which I strive to grow.

For those struggling to conceive, here are a few ways I've learned to respond if thoughtless comments come your way. Keep in mind that these are my opinions, and each person is different. However, I have heard other women in similar situations make suggestions like these.

- Plan standard responses for when those awkward conversations arrive, such as, "We hope to have a baby any time now."

- Begin by telling people you trust that you are having difficulty getting pregnant. Practice with those who are easy to tell and with trusted friends. As you grow more comfortable, you can tell people that you desire to be a mother but that it just hasn't happened yet. We have found that it helps to be up-front with everyone. Then people can pray for us and encourage us, and they won't ask when we're planning to have kids.

- Take a deep breath or pause for a moment, then choose your response carefully. Remind yourself that responding to hurtful words with more hurtful words is not the answer.

- Realize that people are probably trying to encourage you, even when they say things that seem insensitive. Any time that you are able to, receive their words as encouragement. When someone says, "Oh, it will happen," believe those words.

- Receive prayer. If someone says that they will pray for you, then thank them. Don't be afraid to ask people to pray for you.

For those reading this who have not struggled to get pregnant, here are some ways that you can be sensitive to those who are.

- Don't give your opinion on what the couple should or should not be doing. If the couple wants your opinion, they'll ask for it. Otherwise, simply offer a listening ear.

- Don't say: "I hear that if you adopt, you'll get pregnant." Of course, this has happened, but probably more often people adopt but do not get pregnant. I think that the idea behind this is that the woman takes her mind off of her fertility struggle and focuses on the adoption process, and then becomes pregnant because she's "not thinking about it." I could name many couples who have adopted but not become pregnant, and I strongly believe that jumping into the adoption process is not a magic formula that makes someone fertile. I'll address this further in the next chapter.

- Don't say: "Maybe you just need to relax." This is my least favorite! First of all, we were vacationing in Europe when we first started trying to conceive and it was pretty "relaxed" if you ask me. There have been months when my mind has been on other things and I have been quite relaxed, however I did not get pregnant. I personally recognize that I have a very type-A personality and that relaxing is not easy for me, but I'm not convinced that "relaxing" will guarantee pregnancy. I realize that this is well-meant advice, however one reason I don't like this concept of being told to "just relax" is that it seems to places the blame on the woman for not being pregnant because she is not "relaxed" enough.

- Don't say: "Stop thinking about it and it will happen." Although people might really mean "don't obsess about it," telling me to "stop thinking about it" is a comment that I detest. I have been charting my menstrual cycle for so many years that my brain is deeply connected to my fertility. On any given day I know where I am in my cycle, therefore I know if I'm near ovulation, or if I at the time where my periods usually start. My reproductive system speaks in a loud and clear voice to me, therefore it is not easy to "stop thinking about it." I believe that the desire I feel to have a baby is a God-given desire, and although I do all I can to focus on Him throughout this process, I cannot just flip a switch and put my desire for motherhood out of my mind. Trust me – I know that it is really hard not to think about having babies, so my best advice is just to try not to dwell or obsess on it, but to try to take those thoughts captive as I described in Chapter 8.

- Don't suggest sexual positions. Yes, that's how babies come about, however my husband and I don't want anybody else's opinions on that intimate act (nor do we want to imagine you in that particular position). The most common suggestion we hear is for the woman to lay on her back with a pillow elevating her hips after sex. I've been given a few more ideas by well-meaning people, and depending on my mood I've found these recommendations to be either funny or annoying.

- Don't be afraid to tell her that you are pregnant, but do so sensitively. In my years of trying to conceive, I have had friends and family members not want to tell me that they were pregnant since they thought that it might deepen my sadness. The fact is, I like babies, and I like people in my life to have them! Personally, I am more bothered by someone not telling me their good news than by someone gently and kindly telling me that they are expecting. Just make sure that you share the news with sensitivity.

- Don't be afraid to invite her to your baby shower. Maybe it's my imagination, but I have been invited to very few baby showers in the past several years, and I wonder if people have not invited me because they thought that it might cause me sadness. I choose to rejoice for those who rejoice, and I hope that they will one day celebrate with me. I would prefer to be allowed to decline an invitation instead of not being invited at all. But I do realize that some women would rather not be asked than to have to turn down an invitation, since it is too painful for them.

- Try not to complain to your childless friend about your pregnancy or about your children. Realize that women longing for a baby feel like the hardships will be worth it to have a child in their arms. Without a doubt, raising children can be really hard, however I also know what a treasured gift children are.

- Be willing to listen. She may or may not want to talk. There are times that I want to talk about it, and other times I feel too emotional to share. However, I appreciate the people in my life who are willing to listen.

112

Chapter 14 – Why Don't You Just Adopt?

I know the Lord will provide a child for us.
I don't know how and I don't know when.
But I know that He is with us and that He is our God.

Rhonda Rundberg Birchard

Fertility challenges are difficult. There are no easy solutions to the problem, at least for me. At the moment I'm looking back on four years, two surgeries, thousands of dollars, three types of prescription medications, and countless over-the-counter suggestions and home remedies found on the Internet. Of course I wish that I was one of those who could say that we got pregnant right away, but that is obviously not my story.

Often I have wondered if adoption is the route that we should pursue. I've heard it said that "as soon as you adopt you'll get pregnant!" Yes, there are people who adopt and then get pregnant. But there are also many, many people who adopt and do not get pregnant. So I write that statement off as a bunch of baloney – adoption is not a method of tricking your body into becoming pregnant. Plus, God is a God of love and relationship, not one who thrives on "if-thens" and magic. If there were a magic formula then somebody would have figured it out and I wouldn't be writing this book. Instead, God is the One who desires for us to walk with Him, rely on Him, communicate with Him, and trust Him as He transforms us in this challenging process.

I've read about and pondered every adoption possibility I can think of, and Mike and I have weighed our options. Domestic adoption is often slow, expensive, and a risk of heartbreak should a birth mother promise a couple her baby and then change her mind. International adoption involves a lot of paperwork, expense, time, and most often, it does not involve adopting a newborn.

Adoption via foster care starts with fostering a child, and although being a foster parent is something I could see myself doing one day, this approach to adoption would likely be a long, slow process. The first of many steps involves attending the local training program. One hindrance for us personally is the fact that little children aren't as frequently in need of homes as older children. A seminar we attended made it clear that the foster care system is not here to find children for parents; they are seeking parents for children. Although we're technically old enough to be parents of teenagers, like many couples, we dream of starting our family with little ones.

Mike and I relied on my salary during the writing of this book since he was a full-time student. We realize that adoption would dramatically impact our finances, not only with the initial cost, but depending upon the circumstances, it could also potentially affect my ability to earn an income as a nanny.

Embryo adoption is another avenue that I have researched. Many people in past years have had excessive numbers of embryos created in labs for the purpose of in-vitro fertilization. Consequently, the extra embryos remain frozen in labs while the parents try to figure out what to do with them. Once the parents feel that their family is complete, but they have leftover embryos, they must figure out whether to dispose of them or to pass them along to another family. I strongly believe that life begins at conception, therefore those frozen embryos are people. Although they were fertilized in a lab, they were created by God, and simply discarding a tiny young life is not honoring life. I personally believe that embryo adoption – a woman receiving that frozen embryo into her own womb – is a great option. That woman can adopt the embryo, have it implanted, and actually give birth to an adopted baby. Ultimately, like any other type of adoption, I believe it's important to follow God's leadership as we ask Him how He would like to provide.

As I mentioned previously, author Donna VanLiere finally decided to adopt when she realized that her body was not conceiving a baby. She was led to adopt because she felt that the Lord impressed Psalm 113:9 (1984 NIV) on her heart that "He settles the barren woman in her home as a happy mother of children." After one miscarriage and years of trying to conceive a baby, she realized that the Scripture describes a "happy mother of children," not a "happy mother of biological children." For some couples, adoption is ultimately the answer when they cannot conceive.

One of the best articles that I've read about infertility was written by Rhonda Rundberg Birchard on TodaysChristianWoman.com[1]. In this article entitled "Death of a Dream" she writes:

> We know adoption may be the route we need to go in order to have a family. We aren't opposed to adoption; we're just still dealing with the fact that our first dream, to have our own child, is dying. Sometimes you need to heal from the loss of one dream before you can create a new one.

Rhonda ends her article with these powerful, faith-filled words that resonate in my heart:

> I know the Lord will provide a child for us. I don't know how and I don't know when. But I know that He is with us and that He is our God.

Adoption doesn't need to be rushed into. It may or may not be God's direction for someone. Personally, as I type this, I am clinging to the understanding that every woman in the Bible who cried out to God for a baby from her own womb eventually had a baby – even those who seemed too old. So we choose to continue to ask God. Along with that, Mike and I want hearts that are so open to God's direction that if or when He says to adopt then we will be blessed with a child through adoption.

I recently spoke with my friend Mandy Bateman, whose miracle baby was born ten years into her marriage, and she shared with me that she had strongly believed that her promised baby would come from her womb. More than once she and her husband began to pursue adoption, then felt strongly convicted that it was not the route that God intended for them.

Mandy says, "If the Lord told you that you are going to birth a child from your body, don't you dare let anybody tell you otherwise. I don't care what letters follow their name, who they are in ministry, or who they are in authority – you hang onto what GOD told you because that is the final say. End of story."

Mandy shared her story with me as I held her miracle baby in my arms. Although giving birth to her happened nearly a decade later than they had anticipated, this couple now holds their daughter in their arms.

On the flip side, I have met others who are at peace with the fact that adoption was their means by which they started their family. A woman I spoke to who had faced infertility and eventually adopted says that she and her husband often look back and wonder why they didn't adopt sooner. She says that their child, now approaching teen years, is the best child that they could have dreamed of having. For her, adoption was the answer. For some, God has given them such a strong desire to mother the orphans that adoption is an obvious answer.

So if someone were to ask me if adoption is the solution for those who are unable to conceive, I certainly wouldn't be able to give an absolute answer. In some cases yes, in others it would be no. Yet I am not the one to determine that answer – a husband and wife seeking the God who knows what's best for them – that is the answer.

Adoption because someone is called to adopt a child is different than adoption as a solution for infertility. Yes, in the long run, it can provide children for a childless couple and parents to children who need them, but my opinion is that we should each count the cost, seek God's direction, and know for sure that adoption is the route that God has for us.

So as I ponder my options, it's clear that our journey to parenthood has been slow, despite my type-A, take-charge, let's-get-it-done tendencies. I remember those who have gone before me, who have waited longer than I have, and who have trusted in a God who is worth believing in. He is good. His ways are right. His timing is right. So I'm going to keep walking this road, holding my husband's hand, and following the leadership of our God, believing for a happy ending to my story.

Chapter 15 – What Else Can I Do?

May the God of hope
fill you with all joy and peace
as you trust in Him,
so that you may overflow with hope
by the power of the Holy Spirit.
Romans 15:13

Waiting is not easy and it helps to do something during the wait. Here are some common tips for beneficial ways to pass the time while waiting for pregnancy, including things I have done personally. (I am not a medical professional and these are simply my suggestions based on information I have read and things that I have learned.)

Work toward having a healthier body. Make small steps toward eating healthier and exercising more. I struggled to get serious about exercising and losing the twenty pounds I gained as a newlywed. Part of my logic was "why lose weight if I'm just going to gain weight when I'm pregnant?" This is sad, but true! Finally, several years into trying to conceive, Mike and I focused on exercising regularly, eating better, then I lost twenty pounds and began running. Before I knew it, I had signed up to run a half marathon. He also lost weight and began running again. It's true – exercise is a great way to relieve stress – plus, now that I'm approaching 35 and trying to start a family, I realize how much I want to be a fit and active mom that can keep up with her kids for years to come.

Work on your finances. Our long-term goal is that I will be the primary caregiver for our children instead of putting them in daycare. This requires keeping our spending low and preparing to live on less income than many of those around us who have two incomes. Plus, fertility treatments can be very expensive. Whether you need to spend this time working, saving, or paying down debt, do it while you can.

Pursue other dreams. One of the dreams I had tucked away years ago was my dream of writing a book and that dream resurfaced in our season of waiting. I began by writing blog posts about this faith journey, then as I wrote about my fertility struggle combined with the hope that God had poured into my heart, I composed this book. In our wait for babies, Mike and I have traveled extensively, he has completed graduate school, and we have done things we might not have done if we'd had little ones when we had planned.

Develop a heart of gratitude. When I was younger, it was obvious that I naturally tended to be more pessimistic than optimistic. It was easy for me to see the negative side of any situation. In the past several years I have learned to consciously choose to see the good in things. My husband, however, is one who purposefully tries to be continually grateful to God – he is always counting his blessings. He reminds me that we have so much to be thankful for (and we intentionally plan to teach our children that mindset as well). Trying to see things from God's perspective, choosing to see the bright side, and even more so, choosing to thank God for His goodness and for His good gifts in all circumstances will only make things better. Our attitudes will be better, our outlook on life will improve, and therefore this long and difficult season of waiting for a baby will be easier. I've been walking this road for several years, and one key reason I believe that I've been able to have an attitude of hope is by developing a mindset of gratitude.

Draw closer to God. There is no one who understands what we're going through better than our Creator. Our husbands will never fully relate to a woman's heart, and our friends may never understand the ups and the downs of waiting for a baby. Yet God knows us fully and He sees the big picture. He knows why this wait for a baby is taking so long. Psalm 145:9 says that, "The Lord is good to all; He has compassion on all He has made." That is His heart toward us. Turn on music that points your heart toward Him and sing it out loud! Read the Bible; its pages are filled with words of hope and encouragement. Pray because He wants to hear from you – and He wants to speak to you.

Word-of-mouth is crucial for any author to succeed. If you enjoyed this book, please follow me on Facebook or leave a review on Amazon. Even if it's just a sentence or two, it would make all the difference and would be very much appreciated.

About the author:

Betsy lives in the Washington, D.C. area, where she works as a nanny. She and her husband Mike have been married for six years, and they're finding that marriage gets better with each year that passes. Together they enjoy exploring new cities on foot, eating at their favorite Italian restaurants, and doing life as a team. Some of Betsy's favorite things include cuddly babies, good coffee, hot showers, the internet, modern worship music, and a cozy bed. Despite the fact that she sometimes wishes that she lived in the *Little House on the Prairie* days, she is grateful to be living here and now.

You'll find more of her writing here:

www.hopeduringinfertility.com

www.lovethatbetsy.com

www.chixpartyoffive.com

www.facebook.com/hopeduringinfertility

Recommended Resources

Fertility Books:

Taking Charge of Your Fertility, 10th Anniversary Edition: The Definitive Guide to Natural Birth Control, Pregnancy Achievement, and Reproductive Health by Toni Weschler – One of the best resources for understanding your reproductive system and learning to chart your fertility cycles.

The Impatient Woman's Guide to Getting Pregnant by Jean M. Twenge Ph.D. – Of all the fertility books I have read, this one is the most straightforward, concise, and interesting.

How My Soul Yearns: How God Brought Me Through Infertility and Beyond by Ashley Wells – This quick read offers an excellent perspective of hope from a young woman who was told by doctors that she would never be able to conceive outside of God's intervention.

Hannah's Hope: Seeking God's Heart in the Midst of Infertility, Miscarriage, and Adoption Loss by Jennifer Saake – The author writes about what she has learned from her personal experiences. She also shares lessons from Hannah in the Bible.

Every Drunken Cheerleader: Why Not Me? by Kristine Ireland Waits – One woman's story of wrestling through her journey to motherhood.

The Infertility Companion: Hope and Help for Couples Facing Infertility by Sandra L. Glahn and William R. Cutrer – Co-authored by a woman who struggled with infertility and a medical doctor who treated infertility patients, this book offers a balanced perspective. It is endorsed by the Christian Medical Association.

Fertility Resources:

Fertility Friend app – **fertilityfriend.com/** – This can be downloaded as an app on your phone or used through the website fertilityfriend.com. I find it to be very helpful in charting my cycles.

Wondfo Ovulation and Pregnancy Test Strips – Although pharmacies and other retailers offer a variety of ovulation and pregnancy tests, my favorite and least expensive option is the Wondfo brand strips found on Amazon.

Basal Body Temperature Thermometers – I have used this same trusty thermometer for at least five years and can't complain!

Books I Mentioned:

Finding Grace: A True Story About Losing Your Way In Life...And Finding It Again by Donna VanLiere

A Million Little Ways: Uncover the Art You Were Made to Live by Emily P. Freeman

Longing Heart; Empty Arms by Sally M. Jones

Remember the Roses: How to Hold Out, Hang On, and Marry the Man of Your Dreams by Lynette Lewis

The Respect Dare: 40 Days to a Deeper Connection with God and Your Husband by Nina Roesner

More about Restoring the Foundations:

Biblical Healing and Deliverance: A Guide to Experiencing Freedom from Sins of the Past, Destructive Beliefs, Emotional and Spiritual Pain, Curses and Oppression by Chester and Betsy Kylstra (www.rtfi.org)

Notes

Chapter 4: Then Comes the Baby… or Not?

1. Toni Weschler, *Taking Charge of Your Fertility: The Definitive Guide to Natural Birth Control, Pregnancy Achievement, and Reproductive Health (Revised Edition)* (New York, NY: William Morrow Paperbacks, 2006).

Chapter 5: Miracle Babies

1. Nina Roesner, *The Respect Dare: 40 Days to a Deeper Connection with God and Your Husband* (Nashville, TN: Thomas Nelson, 2012).

Chapter 6: It's Not Easy, Yet God is Good

1. http://everybitterthingissweet.com/2014/05/mothers-day-a-day-to-shed-that-thick-skin-a-note-for-the-not-yet-mamas-and-others-in-waiting/

2. http://www.resolve.org/about/fast-facts-about-fertility.html

3. *Hope's Anthem* by William Matthews & Christa Black Gifford http://bethelmusic.com/chords/hopes-anthem/

4. *Prologue to the Fall* by Jon and Kelley Owens http://jonowens.tv/wp-content/uploads/2014/09/Prologue-to-the-Fall.pdf

Chapter 7: I'm Not Alone

1. Donna VanLiere, *Finding Grace: A True Story About Losing Your Way In Life…And Finding It Again* (New York, NY: St. Martin's Press, 2009).

2. http://podcasts.ibethel.org/en/podcasts/birthing-the-impossible

Chapter 8: Thoughts and Words

1. Restoring the Foundations www.rtfi.org

2. Sally M. Jones, *Longing Heart; Empty Arms* (Three Rivers, MI: Ajoyin Publishing, 2013).

3. Emily P. Freeman, *A Million Little Ways: Uncover the Art You Were Made to Live* (Grand Rapids, MI: Baker Publishing, 2013).

Chapter 10: My Crowd of Witnesses

1. http://podcast.kingspark.org/may-11-mothers-day-agony-ecstasy-and-the-boring-in-between-lynette-lewis/

2. Lynette Lewis, *Remember the Roses: How to Hold Out, Hang On, and Marry the Man of Your Dreams* (Franklin, TN: Carpenter's Son Publishing, 2012).

Chapter 14: Why Don't You Just Adopt?

1. http://www.todayschristianwoman.com/articles/2010/april/deathofadream.html

Acknowledgements:

Mike, I am forever grateful that God has knitted us together in marriage. Even before our first date, I sensed God showing me that you would be a good husband and a good father, and I'm grateful that we have such a wonderful marriage! I have loved seeing a glimpse of your father's heart in the way that you love our nieces and nephews and the other children in our lives. Thank you for your unwavering support in my desire to write this book. I am grateful for the time you gave me to focus on writing and for the fact that you supported me through every step. I most definitely appreciate your help in editing the content in this book. There is no one else I'd rather journey through life with than you.

My parents, Liza & David Hopper, thank you for being praying parents! I get my love of children from you, Mom, and am so grateful that you and Dad are my parents! The happy childhood that you gave me, Lydia, Martha, and Tim magnifies my desire to have my own little ones.

My in-laws, Lydia & Jim Herman, thanks for bringing your son into this world! Mom H., I have appreciated your insight as I finalized this manuscript.

Thank you to the Chix for years of emailing back and forth and jumping into the blogging adventure with me! You've each had a vital role in my life and in my book.

Brandy K., thank you for being one of my biggest cheerleaders when I first shared the vision for this book. Thank you for the text messages and emails that kept me writing in those early months. I am grateful for your prayers! Samuel K., thank you for proofreading and editing, giving me valuable perspective.

Bethany P., thank you for putting your hardcore editing skills to work on my rough draft. Your insight and comments made this book better!

Rebekah H., thank you for your encouragement and for creating the beautiful cover during a very busy season!

Julie W., thank you for your prayers. Thank you for telling me several years ago that you thought that I was a good writer – it helped give me the confidence to pursue this.

Charity V., thank you for working so hard as our final editor! I appreciated hearing your perspective, and you encouraged me greatly.

Kim B., your support helped me on many levels – encouraging me in the writing process, editing the manuscript twice, and taking such beautiful photos during a nearly-spontaneous photo shoot!

Thanks to Pasaka, Jennifer, Martha, Mavette, Vonyee, Andrea, Sonya, Mayra, Bethany, Tracy, Lauren, and others for reading my manuscript and sharing your thoughts with me.

Thank you, Meghan, for being a listening ear in the past couple of years.

To Mandy, "Debra," and "Michelle" who allowed me to share their stories of miracle babies: thank you for letting your stories be known. When I see what God has done for you, I believe that He can do it for all of us!

Tom S., thank you for assisting with the back cover text.

To the many friends I have journeyed alongside as you also ask God for babies, I continue to stand with you. Although I won't name you here, I will be cheering "Yes, Yay, and Amen!" when your babies come!

Markus Loacker, thank you for sharing your research and depth of knowledge with marketing. The many hours of help you put into this project have been invaluable. We also appreciate your input with the content of the book. Thanks to you and Heike for encouraging Mike and me through the years!

Thanks to S.K.M. and P.M. for allowing me to love your children each day while I await my own.

To the many families who have entrusted their children into my care over the years, your little ones have been my joy and delight.

Thank you to each person that I mention in this book, especially those who have allowed me to share part of your personal story.

To my "crowd of witnesses" (family and friends) who have believed with us for miracle babies, I am so grateful that you are cheering us on.

NewSong Church Writers' Group and Creative Arts Ministry: You are a church that demonstrates what it means to walk with the Holy Spirit. Thank you for being a safe place for me to share my heart and to birth this book. Grace, thank you for challenging us to bring the hard stuff we're composing into the writers' group. Thank you for being a church that encourages the artists, because you helped to unlock the words and the calling that God has for me as a writer.

Ultimately, I thank God for being the Author of my life's story and the One who I have turned to time and time again through this challenging and painful journey. You, God, are faithful to the end, and in my desire to be more like You, I choose to stand faithful to the end.